Richard Milton Cary

Skirmishers' Drill and Bayonet Exercise

Richard Milton Cary

Skirmishers' Drill and Bayonet Exercise

ISBN/EAN: 9783337130794

Printed in Europe, USA, Canada, Australia, Japan

Cover: Foto ©ninafisch / pixelio.de

More available books at **www.hansebooks.com**

SKIRMISHERS' DRILL

AND

BAYONET EXERCISE

(AS NOW USED IN THE FRENCH ARMY),

WITH

SUGGESTIONS FOR THE SOLDIER IN ACTUAL CONFLICT.

COMPILED AND TRANSLATED

FOR THE USE OF THE VOLUNTEERS OF THE STATE OF VIRGINIA AND THE SOUTH,

BY

R. MILTON CARY,

LT. COL., PROV. ARMY VA.

"The bayonet is the weapon of the brave."

RICHMOND, VA:
WEST & JOHNSTON,
145 MAIN STREET.
1861.

Entered according to Act of Congress, in the year 1861, by
WEST & JOHNSTON,
In the Clerk's Office of the District Court of the Confederate States for the Eastern District of Virginia.

INTRODUCTION.

The accompanying pages have been compiled and translated by the undersigned for the purpose of supplying what he believes an important want to the volunteers of the South.

The self-reliance and personal courage so universal with the people of our country will render them equal to any others in the world, in the capacity of light troops, provided they are properly trained.

This little volume embraces the deployments, rallies, and assemblies of a company of skirmishers, and the drill of the bayonet and sabre-bayonet now in use in the French army, with such suggestions to the soldier in actual conflict as are given by French military writers. Those suggestions, and the exercise for the bayonet, have been taken from the official books of instruction of that most military of all nations; and the instruction for the movements of skirmishers has been taken from the system of tactics prepared by Col. Hardee, late U. S. A. The value of the bayonet exercise is not a matter of speculation. Its practicability is no longer an open question; it has been brought to its present actual efficiency through a succession of trials, all of them improved by practice, first on the drill ground, and then on the battle-field.

It is absolutely necessary for light infantry. If attacked by cavalry, when deployed as skirmishers, they must rely mainly upon their bayonets. It is important that they should understand the great value of the weapon, and the best mode of using it. To show the importance of the weapon, and of instruction in its use, it is deemed not out of place here to give a brief sketch of the origin and progress of such instruction in the French service.

In 1828, the Superior Council of War of France had under discussion the question of abolishing the light infantry; when, instead of doing away with it, a new impetus was given towards promoting its efficiency. After various essays, the formation of a special corps was resolved on, in 1838. The first battalion organized answered so well its purpose, that in 1840 ten battalions of twelve hundred and fifty-nine men each were formed. These are the celebrated "*Chasseurs de Vincennes*" and "*Zouaves*," which are now fourfold their original numbers. The improvements made from time to time have culminated in the adoption of the skirmishers' drill, rifled arms, the sabre-bayonet, and the use of the bayonet according to the principles of fencing, as herein prescribed. The results obtained have been even beyond expectation. From that time the French began to sweep before them the fearless Arabs in Algeria, in spite of their almost fabulous contempt of danger, and excellence in horsemanship.

The Russian infantry in the Crimea, and the Austrian infantry in Lombardy, both equal to any other infantry of the line in the world, each in turn, were over-matched and defeated by the French troops trained in this drill. It will be recollected that the Emperor of the French, at the opening of the campaign in Lombardy, after his landing at Genoa, issued a short and telling proclamation to his soldiers; in it he reminds them that, after all, "they had to rely on their bayonets for the victory;" and this is so much the more significant, that it fell from the lips of one who had endowed his army with the improved Minie rifle, and with those rifled guns of his own invention, which made such havoc amongst the Austrian cavalry at Solferino, and were then without rivals in the field, since the Armstrong gun of the English was not completed, and was only tried in actual service in the late China war.

Notwithstanding all those advantages, Louis Napoleon did not think it out of season to warn his soldiers just before action, that it is for the bayonet to strike the decisive blow. Thus far he seems to agree with another great practical chieftain, the Russian General, Souwarrow, who used to say, in his picturesque language, "The bullet is foolish; the bayonet alone is wise."

These details have been entered into in order that it may be well understood that the drill which this book is intended to introduce to the volunteers of the State and of the South, is not an unimportant work of fancy, contrived for amusement; but, on the contrary, is the fruit of time and experience, rendered into a practical form by military men, who all acknowledge it to be one of the most powerful agencies of modern warfare.

This book is, therefore, nothing but a translation; the plates being *fac-similes* of those obtained from Paris; and the only merit which is claimed for it is, that it renders, in our language, the latest and most approved instruction for the use of the bayonet, in connection with the skirmishers' drill, in a convenient form, and for small cost. The skirmishers' drill and the bayonet drill were intended by their inventors to go together. The one is incomplete in the absence of the other. As bearing upon the skirmishers' drill, we will indulge ourselves with an extract from a very remarkable article published in the "*Moniteur de l'Armee*," in 1851, by a captain of the staff, DuCasse. He says: "It was a noble and admirable idea, that of connecting together four men, neighbors to each other in the ranks, under the name of *comrades in battle*, and to tell them, 'Every one of you is bound for the whole, and upon each devolves the care of preserving the life of the three others.' No measure more apt to foster that noble and brotherly feeling, which in the army is called *esprit de corps*, could have been imagined. The idea of *comrades in battle*, acting in groups for self-defence, forming in the plain to resist cavalry, as many little squares, each element of which is ready to fight to the death in order to protect the life of his brothers in arms, is one of the most successful among those brought forth in the organization of the '*Chasseurs-a-pied*.'

"Called upon, by the special purpose which they answer, to fight nearly always isolated, and not by platoons or battalions, the skirmishers required an individual instruction more thorough than that of the other infantry men.

The ordinance made for them has provided for it; to the regular manual of arms have been added volts, demi-volts, bayonet-fencing, the art of attacking cavalry and resisting their attacks. In short, the service of the skirmishers has been so extended as to become an habitual, not an accidental service; and the men have been enabled to fight in that order the whole day, without rallying upon the platoon or battalion, cases of absolute necessity being excepted."

By the ordinance of July 22, 1845, the skirmishers' drill and bayonet exercise were restricted to the "*Chasseurs;*" but by a ministerial decree of the 7th of April, 1851, they were extended *to all of the infantry* of the French army. The drill which is offered to the volunteers of the South in this book is that now in use by the French infantry as well as the "Chasseurs," and a portion of it was adopted as late as 1858.

The undersigned begs to be indulged in saying that he puts forth this little work with no desire to make money. His object is to place within reach of his fellow-volunteers valuable and important material, in the hope that thereby our efficiency as soldiers may be promoted.

He acknowledges the very valuable assistance of Mons. C. F. Pardigon, a native of Paris (at present attached to the Wise Legion, and a very devoted and true soldier of the Old Dominion), rendered him in getting up and translating the book.

R. M. C.

RICHMOND, VA., July, 1861.

INSTRUCTION FOR SKIRMISHERS.

ARTICLE FIRST.

DEPLOYMENTS.

1. A company may be deployed as skirmishers in two ways: forward, and by the flank.

2. The deployment forward will be adopted when the company is behind the line on which it is to be established as skirmishers; it will be deployed by the flank, when it finds itself already on that line.

3. Whenever a company is to be deployed as skirmishers, it will be divided into two platoons, and each platoon will be subdivided into two sections; the comrades in battle, forming groups of four men, will be careful to know and to sustain each other. The captain will assure himself that the files in the centre of each platoon and section are designated.

4. A company may be deployed as skirmishers on its right, left, or centre file, or on any other named file whatsoever. In this manner, skirmishers may be thrown forward with the greatest possible rapidity on any ground they may be required to occupy.

5. A chain of skirmishers ought generally to preserve their alignment, but no advantages which the ground may present should be sacrificed to attain this regularity.

6. The interval between skirmishers depends on the extent of ground to be covered; but in general, it is not proper that the groups of four men should be removed more than forty paces from each other. The habitual distance between men of the same group, in open grounds, will be five paces; in no case will they lose sight of each other.

TO DEPLOY FORWARD.

7. A company being at a halt, or in march, when the captain shall wish to deploy it forward on the left file of

the first platoon, holding the second platoon in reserve, he will command:

1. *First platoon—As skirmishers.*
2. *On the left file—Take intervals.*
3. MARCH (*or Double quick*—MARCH.)

8. At the first command, the second and third lieutenants will place themselves rapidly two paces behind the centres of the right and left sections of the first platoon; the first corporal (acting as fifth sergeant) will move one pace in front of the centre of the first platoon, and will place himself between the two sections in the front rank as soon as the movement begins; the fourth sergeant will place himself on the left of the front rank of the same platoon, as soon as he can pass. The captain will indicate to this sergeant the point on which he wishes him to direct his march. The first lieutenant, placing himself before the centre of the second platoon, will command:

Second platoon backward—MARCH.

9. At this command, the second platoon will step three paces to the rear, so as to unmask the flank of the first platoon. It will then be halted by its chief, and the second sergeant will place himself on the left, and the third sergeant on the right flank of this platoon.

10. At the command *march*, the left group of four men, conducted by the fourth sergeant, will direct itself on the point indicated; all the other groups of four, throwing forward briskly the left shoulder, will move diagonally to the front in double-quick time, so as to gain to the right the space of twenty paces, which shall be the distance between each group and that immediately on its left. When the second group from the left shall arrive on a line with, and twenty paces from the first, it will march straight to the front, conforming to the gait and direction of the first, keeping constantly on the same alignment and at twenty paces from it. The third group, and all the others, will conform to what has just been prescribed for the second; they will arrive successively on the line. The right guide will arrive with the last group.

DEPLOYMENTS.

11. The left guide having reached the point where the left of the line should rest, the captain will command the skirmishers to halt; the men composing each group of four will then immediately deploy at five paces from each other, and to the right and left of the front rank man of the even file in each group, the rear-rank men placing themselves on the left of their file-leaders. If any groups be not in line at the command *halt*, they will move up rapidly, conforming to what has just been prescribed.

12. If, during the deployment, the line should be fired upon by the enemy, the captain may cause the groups of four to deploy, as they gain their proper distances.

13. The line being formed, the non-commissioned officers on the right, left, and centre of the platoon will place themselves ten paces in rear of the line, and opposite the positions they respectively occupied. The chiefs of sections will promptly rectify any irregularities, and then place themselves twenty-five or thirty paces, in rear of the centre of their sections, each having with him four men taken from the reserve, and also a bugler, who will repeat, if necessary, the signals sounded by the captain. (See Fig. 1.)

14. Skirmishers should be particularly instructed to take advantage of any cover which the ground may offer, and should lie flat on the ground whenever such a movement is necessary to protect them from the fire of the enemy. Regularity in the alignment should yield to this important advantage.

15. When the movement begins, the first lieutenant will face the second platoon *about*, and march it promptly, and by the shortest line, to about one hundred and fifty paces in rear of the centre of the line. He will hold it always at this distance, unless ordered to the contrary.

16. The reserve will conform itself to all the movements of the line. This rule is general.

17. Light troops will carry their bayonets habitually in the scabbard, and this rules applies equally to the skirmishers and the reserve; whenever bayonets are required to be fixed, a particular signal will be given. The captain will give a general superintendence to the whole deployment, and then promptly place himself about eighty

paces in rear of the centre of the line. He will have with him a bugler, and four men taken from the reserve.

18. The deployment may be made on the right or the centre of the platoon, by the same commands, substituting the indication *right* or *centre* for that of *left* file.

19. The deployment on the right or the centre will be made according to the principles prescribed above; in this latter case, the centre of the platoon will be marked by the right group of four in the second section; the first corporal (acting as a file closer) will place himself on the right of this group, and serve as the guide of the platoon during the deployment.

20. In whatever manner the deployment be made, on the right, left, or centre, the men in each group of four will always deploy at five paces from each other, and upon the front-rank man of the even-numbered file. The deployments will habitually be made at twenty paces interval; but if a greater interval be required, it will be indicated in the command.

21. If a company be thrown out as skirmishers so near the main body as to render a reserve unnecessary, the entire company will be extended in the same manner, and according to the same principles, as for the deployment of a platoon. In this case, the third lieutenant will command the fourth section, and a non-commissioned officer, designated for that purpose, the second section; the first corporal will take the place of fourth sergeant, and the second corporal will act as centre guide; the file-closers will place themselves ten paces in rear of the line, and opposite their places in line of battle. The first and second lieutenants will each have a bugler near him.

TO DEPLOY BY THE FLANK.

22. The company being at a halt, when the captain shall wish to deploy it by the flank, holding the first platoon in reserve, he will command:

1. *Second platoon—As skirmishers.*
2. *By the right flank—Take intervals.*
3. MARCH (*or Double quick*—MARCH).

23. At the first command, the first and third lieutenants will place themselves respectively two paces behind the centres of the first and second sections of the second platoon; the first corporal (who will have been placed as a file-closer) will place himself one pace in front of the centre of the second platoon; the third sergeant, as soon as he can pass, will place himself on the right of the front rank of the same platoon; the captain will indicate to him the point on which he wishes him to direct his march. The chief of the first platoon will execute what has been prescribed for the chief of the second platoon, Nos. 8 and 9. The fourth sergeant will place himself on the left flank of the reserve; the first sergeant will remain on the right flank.

24. At the second command, the first and third lieutenants will place themselves two paces behind the left group of their respective sections.

25. At the command *march,* the second platoon will face to the right, and commence the movement; the left group of four will stand fast, but will deploy as soon as there is room on its right, conforming to what has been prescribed, No. 11; the third sergeant will place himself on the left of the right group, to conduct it; the second group will halt at twenty paces from the one on its left, the third group at twenty paces from the second, and so on to the right. As the groups halt, they will face to the enemy, and deploy as has been explained for the left group.

26. The chiefs of sections will pay particular attention to the successive deployments of the groups, keeping near the group about to halt, so as to rectify any errors which may be committed. When the deployment is completed, they will place themselves thirty paces in rear of the centre of their sections, as has been heretofore prescribed. The non-commissioned officers will also place themselves as previously indicated.

27. As soon as the movement commences, the chief of the first platoon, causing it to face about, will move it as indicated No. 15.

28. The deployment may be made by the left flank according to the same principles, by substituting *left flank* for *right flank.*

29. If the captain should wish to deploy the company upon the centre of one of the platoons, he will command:

1. *Second platoon*—As skirmishers.
2. *By the right and left flanks*—Take intervals.
3. March (or *Double quick*—March.)

30. At the first command, the officers and non-commissioned officers will conform to what has been prescribed, No. 23.

31. At the second command, the first lieutenant will place himself behind the left group of the right section of the second platoon, the third lieutenant behind the right group of the left section of the same platoon.

32. At the command *march*, the right section will face to the right, the left section will face to the left, the group on the right of this latter section will stand fast. The two sections will move off in opposite directions; the third sergeant will place himself on the left of the right file to conduct it, the second sergeant on the right of the left file. The two groups nearest that which stands fast will each halt at twenty paces from this group, and each of the other groups will halt at twenty paces from the group which is in rear of it. Each group will deploy as heretofore prescribed, No. 25.

33. The first and third lieutenants will direct the movement, holding themselves always abreast of the group which is about to halt.

34. The captain can cause the deployment to be made on any named group whatsoever; in this case, the first corporal will place himself before the group indicated, and the deployment will be made according to the principles heretofore prescribed.

35. The entire company may be also deployed according to the same principles.

TO EXTEND INTERVALS.

36. This movement, which is to be employed to extend a line of skirmishers, will be executed according to the principles prescribed for deployments.

37. If it be supposed that the line of skirmishers is

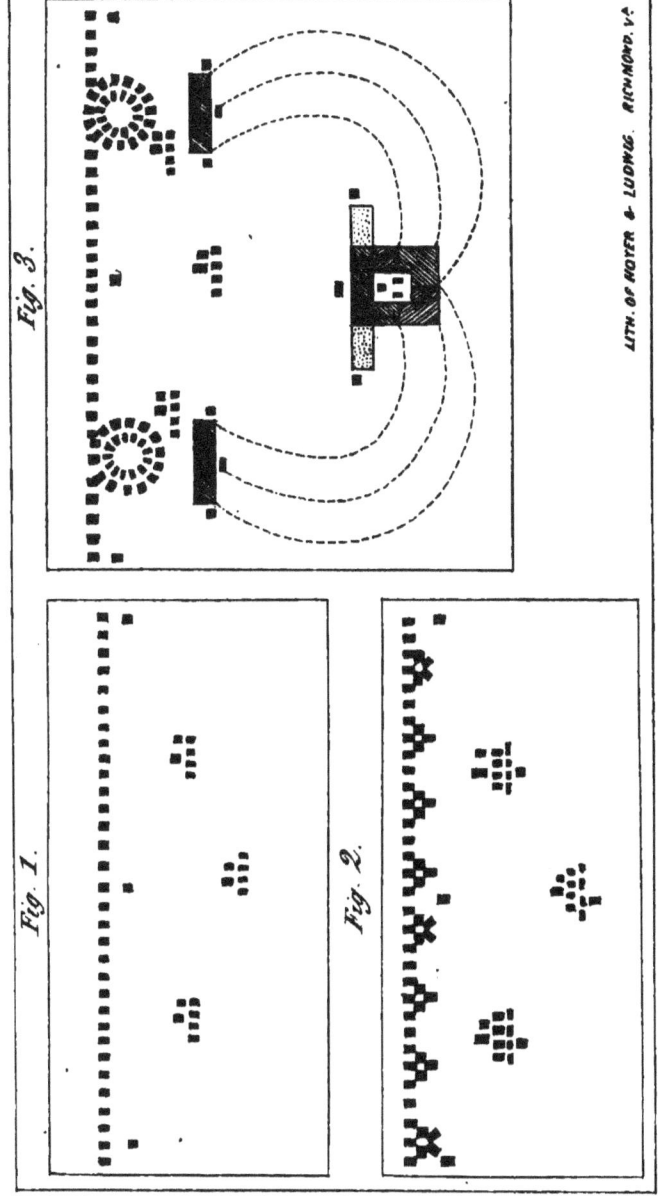

at a halt, and that the captain wishes to extend it to the left, he will command :

1. *By the left flank (so many paces)*—EXTEND INTERVALS.
2. MARCH (or *Double quick*—MARCH).

38. At the command *march*, the group on the right will stand fast, all the other groups will face to the left, and each group will extend its interval to the prescribed distance by the means indicated, No. 25.

39. The men of the same group will continue to preserve between each other the distance of five paces, unless the nature of the ground should render it necessary that they should close nearer in order to keep in sight of each other. The intervals refer to the spaces between the groups, and not to the distances between the men in each group. The intervals will be taken from the right or left man of the neighboring group.

40. If the line of skirmishers be marching to the front, and the captain should wish to extend it to the right, he will command :

1. *On the left group (so many paces)*—EXTEND INTERVALS.
2. MARCH (or *Double quick*—MARCH).

41. The left group, conducted by the guide, will continue to march on the point of direction; the other groups, throwing forward the left shoulder, and taking the double quick step, will open their intervals to the prescribed distance by the means indicated, No. 18, conforming also to what is prescribed, No. 39.

42. Intervals may be extended on the centre of the line, according to the same principles.

43. If, in extending intervals, it be intended that one company or platoon should occupy a line which had been previously occupied by two, the men of the company or platoon which is to retire will fall successively to the rear as they are relieved by the extension of the intervals.

TO CLOSE INTERVALS.

44. This movement, like that of opening intervals, will be executed according to the principles prescribed for the deployments.

45. If the line of skirmishers be halted, and the captain should wish to close intervals to the left, he will command:

1. *By the left flank (so many paces)—Close intervals.*
2. MARCH (*or Double quick—*MARCH).

46. At the command march, the left group will stand fast; the other groups will face to the left and close to the prescribed distance; each group facing to the enemy as it attains its proper distance.

47. If the line be marching to the front, the captain will command:

1. *On the left group (so many paces)—close intervals.*
2. MARCH (*or Double quick—*MARCH).

48. The left group, conducted by the guide, will continue to move on in the direction previously indicated; the other groups, advancing the right shoulder, will close to the left, until the intervals are reduced to the prescribed distance.

49. Intervals may be closed on the right, or on the centre, according to the same principles.

ARTICLE SECOND.

TO ADVANCE.

TO ADVANCE IN LINE, AND TO RETREAT IN LINE.

50. When a platoon or a company, deployed as skirmishers, is marching by the front, the guide will be habitually in the centre. No particular indication to this effect need be given in the commands; but if, on the contrary, it be intended that the directing guide should be

on the right or left, the command, *guide right*, or *guide left*, will be given immediately after that of forward.

51. The captain, wishing the line of skirmishers to advance, will command:
   1. *Forward.*
   2. March (*or Double quick*—March).

52. This command will be repeated with the greatest rapidity by the chiefs of sections, and, in case of need, by the sergeants. This rule is general, whether the skirmishers march by the front or by the flank.

53. At the first command, three sergeants will move briskly on the line, the first on the right, the second on the left, and the third in the centre.

54. At the command *march*, the line will move to the front, the guide charged with the direction will move on the point indicated to him, the skirmishers will hold themselves aligned on this guide, and preserve their intervals towards him.

55. The chiefs of sections will march immediately behind their sections, so as to direct their movements.

56. The captain will give a general superintendence to the movement.

57. When he shall wish to halt the skirmishers, he will command:

Halt.

58. At this command, briskly repeated, the line will halt. The chiefs of sections will promptly rectify any irregularity in the alignment and intervals, and after taking every possible advantage which the ground may offer for protecting the men, they, with the three sergeants in the line, will retire to their proper places in rear.

59. The captain, wishing to march the skirmishers in retreat, will command:
   1. *In retreat.*
   2. March (*or Double quick*—March).

60. At the first command, the three sergeants will move on the line, as prescribed No. 53.

61. At the command *march*, the skirmishers will face about individually, and march to the rear, conforming to the principles prescribed No. 54.

62. The officers and sergeants will use every exertion to preserve order.

63. To halt the skirmishers, marching in retreat, the captain will command:

HALT.

64. At this command, the skirmishers will halt, and immediately face to the front.

65. The chiefs of sections and the three guides will each conform himself to what is prescribed No. 58.

TO CHANGE DIRECTION.

66. If the commander of a line of skirmishers shall wish to cause it to change direction to the right, he will command:

1. *Right wheel.*
2 MARCH (*or Double quick* MARCH).

67. At the command *march*, the right guide will mark time in his place; the left guide will move in a circle to the right, and that he may properly regulate his movements, will occasionally cast his eyes to the right, so as to observe the direction of the line, and the nature of the ground to be passed over. The centre guide will also march in a circle to the right, and in order to conform his movements to the general direction, will take care that his steps are only half the length of the steps of the guide on the left.

68. The skirmishers will regulate the length of their steps by their distance from the marching flank, being less as they approach the pivot, and greater as they are removed from it; they will often look to the marching flank, so as to preserve the direction and their intervals.

69. When the commander of the line shall wish to resume the direct march, he will command:

1. *Forward.* 2. MARCH.

70. At the command *march*, the line will cease to wheel, and the skirmishers will remove direct to the front; the centre guide will march on the point which will be indicated to him.

71. If the captain should wish to halt the line, in place of moving it to the front, he will command:

HALT.

72. At this command the line will halt.

73. A change of direction to the left will be made according to the same principles, and by inverse means.

74. A line of skirmishers marching in retreat, will change direction by the same means, and by the same commands, as a line marching in advance; for example, if the captain should wish to refuse his left, now become the right, he will command: 1. *Left Wheel.* 2. MARCH. At the command *halt*, the skirmishers will face to the enemy.

75. But if, instead of halting the line, the captain should wish to continue to march it in retreat, he will, when he judges the line has wheeled sufficiently, command:

1. *In retreat.* 2. MARCH.

TO MARCH BY THE FLANK.

76. The captain, wishing the skirmishers to march by the right flank, will command:

1. *By the right flank.*
2. MARCH (*or Double quick*—MARCH).

77. At the first command, the three sergeants will place themselves on the line.

78. At the command *march*, the skirmishers will face to the right and move off; the right guide will place himself by the side of the leading man on the right, to conduct him, and will march on the point indicated; each skirmisher will take care to follow exactly in the direction of the one immediately preceding him, and to preserve his distance.

79. The skirmishers may be marched by the left flank, according to the same principles, and by the same

commands, substituting *left* for *right;* the left guide will place himself by the side of the leading man, to conduct him.

80. If the skirmishers be marching by the flank, and the captain should wish to halt them, he will command:

HALT.

81. At this command, the skirmishers will halt and face to the enemy. The officers and sergeants will conform to what has been prescribed No. 58.

82. The reserve should execute all the movements of the line, and be held always about one hundred and fifty paces from it, so as to be in position to second its operations.

83. When the chief of the reserve shall wish to march it in advance, he will command: 1. *Platoon forward.* 2. *Guide left.* 3. MARCH. If he should wish to march it in retreat, he will command: 1. *In retreat.* 2. MARCH. 3. *Guide right.* At the command *halt,* it will re-face to the enemy.

84. The men should be made to understand that the signals or commands, such as *forward,* mean that the skirmishers shall march on the enemy; *in retreat,* that they shall retire; and to *the right or left flank,* that the men must face to the right or left, whatever may be their position.

85. If the skirmishers be marching by the flank, and the captain should wish to change direction to the right (or left), he will command: 1. *By file right* (or *left*). 2. MARCH.

ARTICLE THIRD.

THE FIRINGS.

86. Skirmishers will fire either at a halt or marching.

TO FIRE AT A HALT.

87. To cause this fire to be executed, the captain will command:

Commence—FIRING.

88. At this command, briskly repeated, the men of the front rank will commence firing; they will reload rapidly, and hold themselves in readiness to fire again. During this time the men of the rear rank will come to a ready, and as soon as their respective file leaders have loaded, they will also fire and reload. The men of each file will thus continue the firing, conforming to this principle—that the one or the other shall always have his piece loaded.

89. Light troops should be always calm, so as to aim with accuracy; they should, moreover, endeavor to estimate correctly the distances between themselves and the enemy to be hit, and thus be enabled to deliver their fire with the greater certainty of success.

90. Skirmishers will not remain in the same place whilst reloading, unless protected by accidents in the ground.

TO FIRE MARCHING.

91. This fire will be executed by the same commands as the fire at a halt.

92. At the command *commence firing*, if the line be advancing, the front-rank man of every file will halt, fire, and reload before throwing himself forward. The rear-rank man of the same file will continue to march, and after passing ten or twelve paces beyond his front-rank man, will halt, come to a ready, select his object, and fire when his front-rank man has loaded; the fire will thus continue to be executed by each file; the skirmishers will keep united, and endeavor, as much as possible, to preserve the general direction of the alignment.

93. If the line be marching in retreat, at the command *commence firing*, the front-rank man of every file will halt, face to the enemy, fire, and then reload whilst moving to the rear; the rear-rank man of the same file will continue to march, and halt ten or twelve paces beyond his front-rank man, face about, come to a ready, and fire when his front-rank man has passed him in retreat and loaded; after which, he will move to the rear and reload; the front-rank man, in his turn, after marching briskly to the rear, will halt at ten or twelve paces from the rear-rank,

face to the enemy, load his piece, and fire, conforming to what has just been prescribed; the firing will thus be continued.

94. If the company be marching by the right flank, at the command *commence firing*, the front-rank man of every file will face to the enemy, step one pace forward, halt, and fire; the rear-rank man will continue to move forward. As soon as the front-rank man has fired, he will place himself briskly behind his rear-rank man, and reload whilst marching. When he has loaded, the rear-rank man will, in his turn, step one pace forward, halt, and fire, and returning to the ranks will place himself behind his front-rank man; the latter, in his turn, will act in the same manner, observing the same principles. At the command *cease firing*, the men of the rear-rank will retake their original positions, if not already there.

95. If the company be marching by the left flank, the fire will be executed according to the same principles, but in this case, it will be the rear-rank men who will fire first.

96. The following rules will be observed in the cases to which they apply.

97. If the line be firing at a halt, or whilst marching by the flank, at the command *forward—march*, it will be the men whose pieces are loaded, without regard to the particular rank to which they belong, who will move to the front. Those men whose pieces have been discharged, will remain in their places to load them before moving forward, and the firing will be continued agreeably to the principles prescribed No. 92.

98. If the line be firing either at a halt, advancing, or whilst marching by the flank, at the command *in retreat —march*, the men whose pieces are loaded will remain faced to the enemy, and will fire in this position; the men whose pieces are discharged will retreat loading them; and the fire will be continued agreeably to the principles prescribed No. 93.

99. If the line of skirmishers be firing either at a halt, advancing, or in retreat, at the command, *by the right* (or *left*) *flank*—MARCH, the men whose pieces are loaded will

step one pace out of the general alignment, face to the enemy, and fire in this position; the men whose pieces are unloaded will face to the right (or left), and march in the direction indicated. The men who stepped out of the ranks will place themselves, immediately after firing, upon the general direction, and in rear of their front or rear rank men, as the case may be. The fire will be continued according to the principles prescribed No. 94.

100. Skirmishers will be habituated to load their pieces whilst marching; but they will be enjoined to halt always an instant, when in the act of charging cartridge and priming.

101. They should be practiced to fire and load kneeling, lying down, and sitting, and much liberty should be allowed in these exercises, in order that they may be executed in the manner found to be most convenient. Skirmishers should be cautioned not to forget that, in whatever position they may load, it is important that the piece should be placed upright before ramming, in order that the entire charge of powder may reach the bottom of the bore.

102. In commencing the fire, the men of the same rank should not all fire at once, and the men of the same file should be particular that one or the other of them be always loaded.

103. In retreating, the officer commanding the skirmishers should seize on every advantage which the ground may present, for arresting the enemy as long as possible.

104. At the signal to *cease firing*, the captain will see that the order is promptly obeyed; but the men who may not be loaded will load. If the line be marching, it will continue the movement; but the man of each file who happens to be in front will wait until the man in rear shall be abreast with him.

105. If a line of skirmishers be firing advancing, at the command *halt*, the line will re-form upon the skirmishers who are in front; when the line is retreating, upon the skirmishers who are in rear.

ARTICLE FOURTH.

THE RALLY.—TO FORM COLUMN.

106. A company deployed as skirmishers, is rallied in order to oppose the enemy with better success; the rallies are made at a run, and with bayonets fixed; when ordered to rally, the skirmishers fix bayonets without command.

107. There are several ways of rallying, which the chief of the line will adopt according to circumstances.

108. If the line, marching, or at a halt, be merely disturbed by scattered horsemen, it will not be necessary to fall back on the reserve, but the captain will cause bayonets to be fixed. If the horsemen should, however, advance to charge the skirmishers, the captain will command, *rally by fours.* The line will halt if marching, and the four men of each group will execute this rally in the following manner: the front-rank man of the even-numbered file will take the position of *guard against cavalry;* the rear-rank man of the odd-numbered file will also take the position of *guard against cavalry,* turning his back to him, his right foot thirteen inches from the right foot of the former, and parallel to it; the front-rank man of the odd file, and the rear-rank man of the even file, will also place themselves back to back, taking a like position, and between the two men already established, facing to the right and left; the right feet of the four men will be brought together, forming a square, and serving for mutual support. (See plate 2, pages 8 and 9.) The four men in each group will come to a ready, fire as occasion may offer, and load without moving their feet.

109. The captain and chiefs of sections will each cause the four men who constitute his guard to form square, the men separating so as to enable him and the bugler to place themselves in the centre. The three sergeants will each promptly place himself in the group nearest him in the line of skirmishers.

110. Whenever the captain shall judge these squares

too weak, but should wish to hold his position by strengthening his line, he will command:

Rally by—SECTIONS.—(Plate 8, pages 8 and 9.)

111. At this command, the chiefs of sections will move rapidly on the centre group of their respective sections, or on any other interior group whose position might offer a shelter, or other particular advantage; the skirmishers will collect rapidly, at a run, on this group, without distinction of numbers. The men composing the group on which the formation is made, will immediately form square, as heretofore explained, and elevate their pieces, the bayonets uppermost, in order to indicate the point on which the rally is to be made. The other skirmishers, as they arrive, will occupy and fill the open angular spaces, between these four men, and successfully rally around this first nucleus, and in such manner as to form rapidly a compact circle. The skirmishers will take, as they arrive, the position of charge bayonet, the point of the bayonet more elevated, and will cock their pieces in this position. The movement concluded, the two exterior ranks will fire as occasion may offer, and load without moving their feet.

112. The captain will move rapidly, with his guard, wherever he may judge his presence most necessary.

113. The officers and sergeants will be particular to observe that the rally is made in silence, and with promptitude and order; that some pieces in each of their subdivisions be at all times loaded, and that the fire is directed on those points only where it will be most effective.

114. If the reserve should be threatened, it will form into a circle around its chief.

115. If the captain or commander of a line of skirmishers formed of many platoons, should judge that the rally by section does not offer sufficient resistance, he will cause the rally by platoons to be executed, and for this purpose, will command:

Rally by—PLATOONS.

116. This movement will be executed according to the same principles, and by the same means, as the rally by

sections. The chiefs of platoon will conform to what has been prescribed for the chiefs of sections.

117. The captain wishing to rally the skirmishers on the reserve, will command:

Rally on the—RESERVE.

118. At this command, the captain will move briskly on the reserve; the officer who commands it will take immediate steps to form square; for this purpose, he will cause the half sections on the flanks to be thrown perpendicularly to the rear; he will order the men to come to a ready.

119. The skirmishers of each section, taking the run, will form rapidly into groups, and upon that man of each group who is nearest the centre of the section. These groups will direct themselves diagonally towards each other, and in such manner as to form into sections with the greatest possible rapidity while moving to the rear; the officers and sergeants will see that this formation is made in proper order, and the chiefs will direct their sections upon the reserve, taking care to unmask it to the right and left. As the skirmishers arrive, they will continue and complete the formation of the square begun by the reserve, closing in rapidly upon the latter, without regard to their places in line; they will come to a ready without command, and fire upon the enemy; which will also be done by the reserve as soon as it is unmasked by the skirmishers.

120. If a section should be closely pressed by cavalry while retreating, its chief will command *halt;* at this command, the men will form rapidly into a compact circle around the officer, who will re-form his section and resume the march, the moment he can do so with safety.

121. The formation of the square in a prompt and efficient manner, requires coolness and activity on the part of both officers and sergeants.

122. The captain will also profit by every moment of respite which the enemy's cavalry may leave him; as soon as he can, he will endeavor to place himself beyond the reach of their charges, either by gaining a position where he may defend himself with advantage, or by returning

to the corps to which he belongs. For this purpose, being in square, he will cause the company to break into column by platoons at half distance;' to this effect, he will command:

1. *Form Column.* 2. MARCH.

123. At the command *march*, each platoon will dress on its centre, and the platoon which was facing to the rear will face about without command. The guides will place themselves on the right and left of their respective platoons; those of the second platoon will place themselves at half distance from those of the first, counting from the rear rank. These dispositions being made, the captain can move the column in whatever direction he may judge proper.

124. If he wishes to march it in retreat, he will command:

1. *In Retreat.*
2. MARCH (*or Double quick*—MARCH).

125. At the command *march*, the column will immediately face by the rear rank, and move off in the opposite direction. As soon as the column is in motion, the captain will command:

3. *Guide right* (*or left*).

126. He will indicate the direction to the leading guide; the guides will march at their proper distances, and the men will keep aligned.

127. If again threatened by cavalry, the captain will command:

1. *Form Square.* 2. MARCH.

128. At the command *march*, the column will halt;. the first platoon will face about briskly, and the outer half-sections of each platoon will be thrown perpendicularly to the rear, so as to form the second and third fronts of the square. The officers and sergeants will promptly rectify any irregularities which may be committed.

129. If he should wish to march the column in advance, the captain will command:

1. *Form Column.* 2. MARCH.

130. Which will be executed as prescribed No. 123.

131. The column being formed, the captain will command:

1. *Forward.*
2. March (*or Double quick*—March.)
3. *Guide left* (*or right.*)

132. At the second command, the column will move forward, and at the third command, the men will take the touch of elbows to the side of the guide.

133. If the captain should wish the column to gain ground to the right or left, he will do so by rapid wheels to the side opposite the guide, and for this purpose, will change the guide whenever it may be necessary.

134. If a company be in column by platoon, at half distance, right in front, the captain can deploy the first platoon as skirmishers by the means already explained; but if it should be his wish to deploy the second platoon forward on the centre file, leaving the first platoon in reserve, he will command:

1. *Second platoon—As skirmishers.*
2. *On the centre file—Take intervals.*
3. March (*or Double quick*—March.)

135. At the first command, the chief of the first platoon will caution his platoon to stand fast; the chiefs of sections of the second platoon will place themselves before the centres of their sections; the first corporal, acting as a sergeant, will place himself one pace in front of the centre of the second platoon.

136. At the second command, the chief of the right section, second platoon, will command: *Section right face;* the chief of the left section: *Section left face.*

137. At the command *march*, these sections will move off briskly in opposite directions; and having unmasked the first platoon, the chiefs of sections will respectively command: *By the left flank*—March, and *By the right flank*—March; and as soon as these sections arrive on the alignment of the first platoon, they will command, *As skirmishers*—March. The groups will then deploy, according to prescribed principles, on the right group of the

left section, which will be directed by the first corporal on the point indicated.

138. If the captain should wish the deployment made by the flank, the second platoon will be moved to the front by the means above stated, and halted after passing some steps beyond the alignment of the first platoon; the deployment will then be made by the flank, according to the principles prescribed.

THE ASSEMBLY.

139. A company deployed as skirmishers will be assembled when there is no longer danger of its being disturbed; the assembly will be made habitually in quick time.

140. The captain wishing to assemble the skirmishers on the reserve, will command:

Assemble on the Reserve.

141. At this command the skirmishers will assemble by groups of four; the front-rank men will place themselves behind their rear-rank men; and each group of four will direct itself on the reserve, where each will take its proper place in the ranks. When the company is re-formed, it will rejoin the battalion to which it belongs.

142. It may be also proper to assemble the skirmishers on the centre, or on the right or left of the line, either marching or at a halt.

143. If the captain should wish to assemble them on the centre while marching, he will command:

Assemble on the Centre.

144. At this command, the centre guide will continue to march directly to the front on the point indicated; the front-rank man of the directing file will follow the guide, and be covered by his rear-rank man; the other two comrades of this group, and likewise those on their left, will march diagonally, advancing the left shoulder and accelerating the gait, so as to reform the groups while drawing nearer and nearer the directing file; the men of the right section will unite in the same manner into groups, and

then upon the directing file, throwing forward the right shoulder. As they successively unite on the centre, the men will bring their pieces to the right shoulder.

145. To assemble on the right or left file will be executed according to the same principles.

146. The assembly of a line marching in retreat will also be executed according to the same principles, the front-rank men marching behind their rear-rank men.

147. To assemble the line of skirmishers at a halt, and on the line they occupy, the captain will give the same commands; the skirmishers will face to the right or left, according as they should march by the right or left flank, re-form the groups while marching, and thus arrive on the file which served as the point of formation. As they successively arrive, the skirmishers will support arms.

BAYONET EXERCISE,

WITH THE MUSKET AND THRUST BAYONET.

Part First.

In teaching this exercise the men, if few in number, may be placed in one rank, if more numerous, say exceeding eight or ten, they should be placed in two ranks, in quincons (the second rank showing between the intervals of the first rank). To do this, the instructor, having opened the ranks to four paces, commands:

1. *By the left flank, at four paces, take intervals.*
2. *Quick*—MARCH.

At this command, number one in the first rank stands fast, number one in the rear rank moves two paces to the left, and all of the men in each rank, take the intervals of four paces, moving for that purpose to the left, halt, and face to the front. Intervals can be taken by the right flank by inverse means, and by the same command,

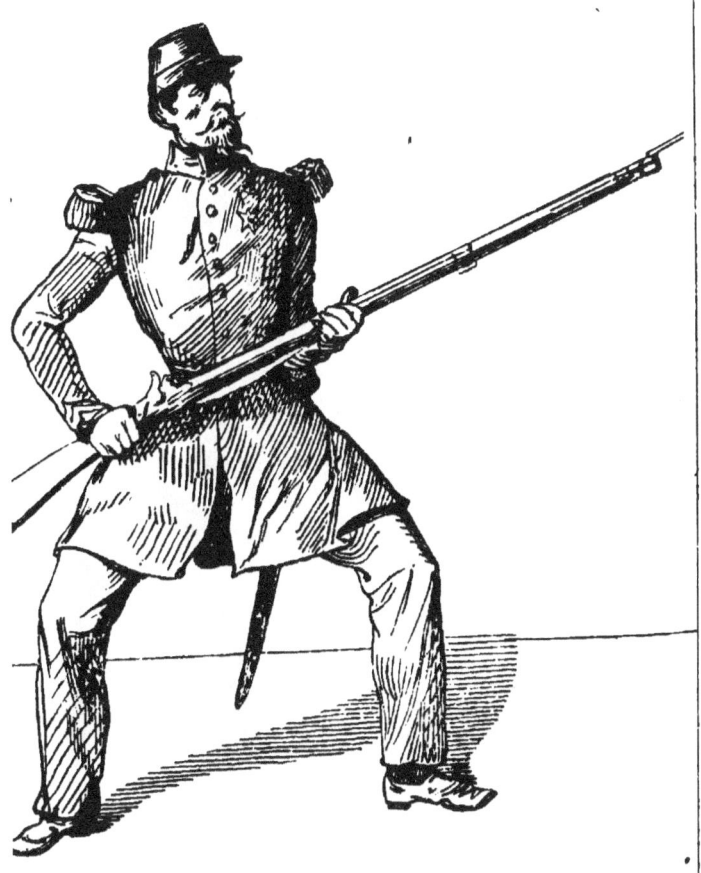

Fig. 1.

Position of the Guard.

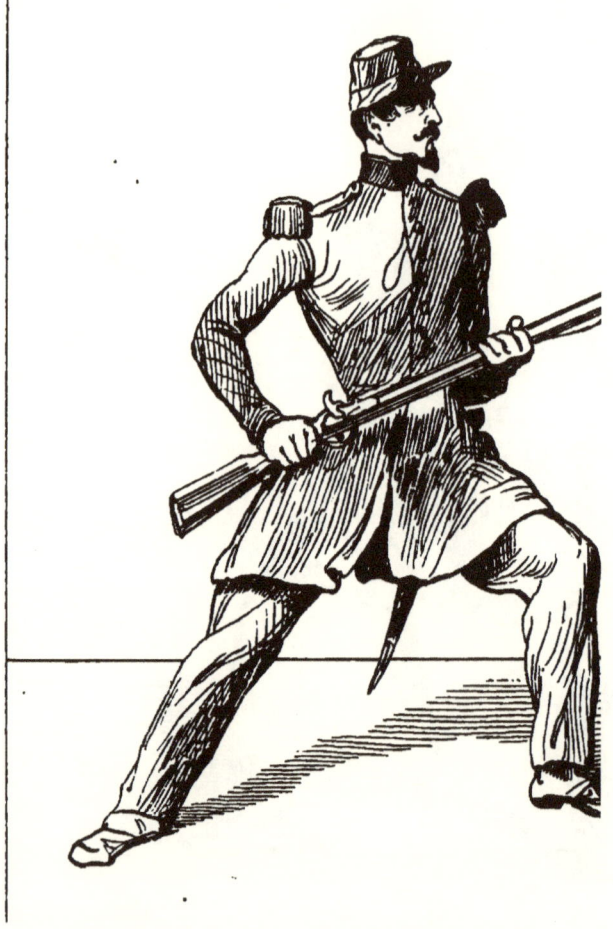

Fig. 2.

Extension.

substituting right for left. To close the ranks and intervals, the instructor commands:

1. *Assemble on No.* 1 (*or any other No.*) *of the front rank.*
2. *Quick*—MARCH.

FIRST LESSON.

SIMPLE MOTIONS.—POSITION OF THE GUARD.

On Guard. (*Two motions.*) (Fig. 1.)

1. Being at a light infantry shoulder, raise a little the piece with the right hand, turn the left toe square to the front.
2. Carry the right foot about eighteen inches backward, the right heel on the prolongation of the left, the body erect and perpendicular on both legs, so that the weight is divided equally between them, the knees bent, and take the position of charge bayonet.

At the command, *shoulder arms,* spring the musket up into the hollow of the right shoulder, and retake the position of the soldier.

The instructor, wishing to allow a rest, when recruits are on guard, commands *Rest.*

At this command, the man brings the right foot by the side of the left, places the butt of the musket on the ground, and is no longer required to remain immovable or to preserve silence.

The instructor, wishing to resume the position of guard, commands:

1. *Attention—Squad* (*or Platoon*).
2. *Resume*—GUARD.

At this command, raise the piece quickly with the right hand, seizing it with the left, at the height of the right breast, and at the same time grasp the small of the stock with the right hand, taking the guard, as before explained.

EXTENSION.

Extend—MARCH. (*One motion.*) (Fig. 2.)

At the second command advance quickly the left foot about twelve inches, the left leg (from knee to ankle) vertical, the right foot flat on the ground, and the right leg extended and straight, the body remaining erect.

At the command, *on guard*, retake the position of guard, by bringing back the left foot to its former position.

1. *Face to the right (or left.)*
2. *Right (or left)*—FACE. (*One motion.*)

Turn on the left heel, raising a little the toe of that foot; face to the right (or left), and carry at the same time the right foot eighteen inches to the rear.

1. *Face about to the right (or left.)*
2. *Right (or left) about*—FACE. (*One motion.*)

Turn to the right (or left) on the left heel, by raising the toe of the left foot, facing to the rear, without changing position of the piece, carrying the right foot eighteen inches to rear, and keeping the body erect.

1. *One pace forward*—MARCH. (*Two motions.*)

1st motion: Carry first the right foot against the left heel.

2d motion: Advance the left foot about eighteen inches, preserving the position of the piece and the body.

1. *One pace backward*—MARCH. (*Two motions.*)

1. Bring back the left foot against the right.
2. Then carry the right foot eighteen inches to the rear.

1. *One pace to the right*—MARCH. (*Two motions.*)

1st motion: Carry the foot about eighteen inches to the right in the same direction.

2d motion: Bring immediately the left foot the same distance, and to the same relative position to the right, that it before occupied.

1. *One pace to the left*—MARCH. (*Two motions.*)

1st motion: Carry the left foot about eighteen inches to the left.

2d motion: Bring back immediately the right foot at its distance, and in its position.

Passade forward—MARCH. (*Two motions.*)

1st motion: Throw the right foot eighteen inches in front of the left, the inside of it kept to the front.

2d motion: Carry quickly the left foot eighteen inches in front of the right, preserving the guard.

Passade backward—MARCH. (*Two motions.*)

1st motion: Throw the left foot eighteen inches in rear of the right foot.

2d motion: Carry quickly the right foot eighteen inches in rear of the left, preserving the guard.

Leap to the rear—MARCH. (*One motion.*)

Throw the weight of the body on the left leg, and spring backward as far as possible, preserving the guard.

1. *Volt to the right*—MARCH. (*Two motions.*)

1st motion: Raise the piece by bringing the left hand near to the left breast, without moving the right, the barrel turned toward the body, and at same time turn to the right on the toe of the right foot, carrying the left foot to its place and distance.

2d motion: Turn to the right on the toe of the left foot; carry the right to its place and distance, at the same time resuming the guard.

Volt to the left—MARCH. (*Two motions.*)

1st motion: Bring the piece to the position last explained; turn to the left on the toe of the right foot, carrying the left to its place and distance.

2d motion: Turn to the left on the toe of the left foot, carrying the right to its place and distance, and resume guard.

SECOND LESSON.

PARRIES.*

Tierce (or three) designates the parry to the right in the upper line.

Carte (or four), the parry to the left in the upper line.

Seconde (or two) designates the parry to the right in lower line.

Prime (or one), the parry to the left in the lower line.

The upper line comprehends that portion of the body above the waist. The lower line, that portion below the waist.

Parry three—ARMS.   (*Two motions.*)   (Fig. 3.)

1. Move the piece six inches to the right, with the left hand, without changing the position of the right hand.
2. Resume guard.

Parry four—ARMS.   (*Two motions.*)   (Fig. 4.)

1. Move the piece to the left, about six inches, with the left hand, moving the right hand slightly to the left around the hip.
2. Resume guard.

Parry one—ARMS.   (*Two motions.*)   (Fig. 5.)

1. Turn rapidly the rammer of the piece upward; describe a half circle with the point of the bayonet from above to below, to throw the piece of the adversary outside of the line of the left knee; bring the left elbow near to the side, the right hand at the height of the forehead, opposite to and six inches from the right eye.
2. Resume guard.

---

* In fencing with the bayonet, the men are considered as right-handed, although the body is faced to the right, and the left knee and left shoulder are foremost. The fact is, the left hand is auxiliary only, the right hand governing the piece.

Therefore the man parries *tierce* (parry three) when he throws the piece of his adversary to his own right, and parries *carte* (parry four) when he throws the piece of his adversary to his own left. In the line below the waist, the *prime* parry (parry one) corresponds to parry four in the line above the waist; and *seconde* parry (parry two) corresponds to parry three in that (the upper) line.

Fig. 3.

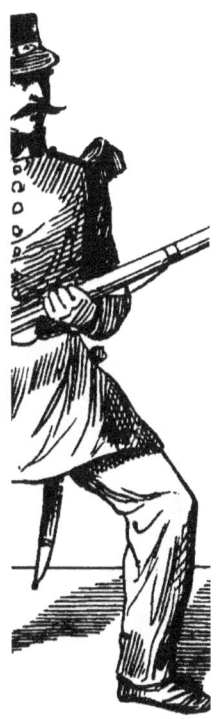

Parry three.

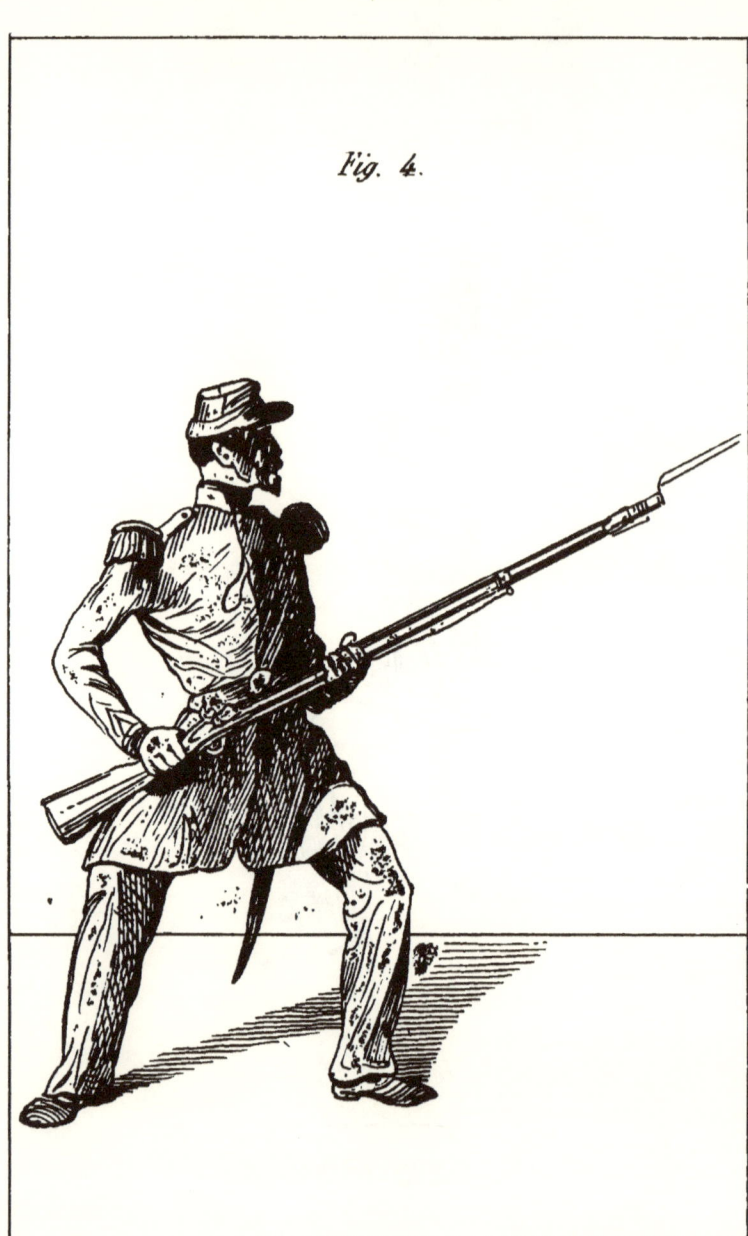

Fig. 4.

Parry four.

Fig. 5.

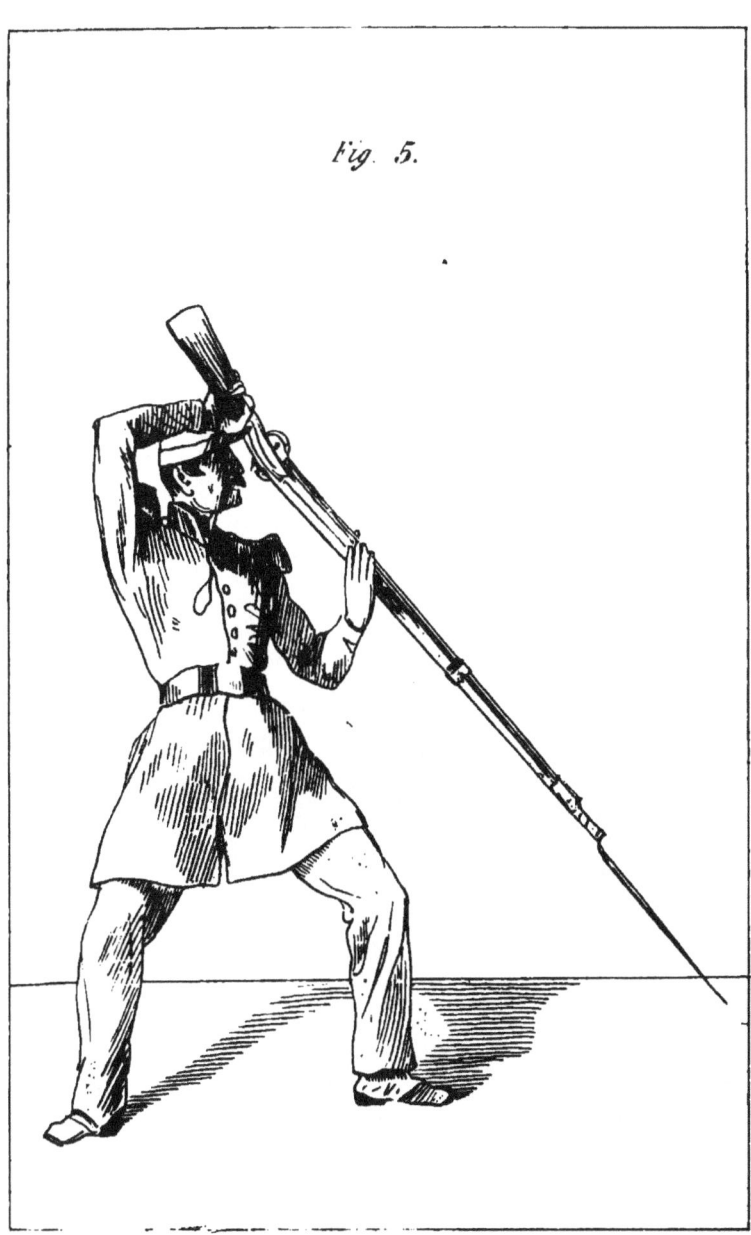

Parry one.

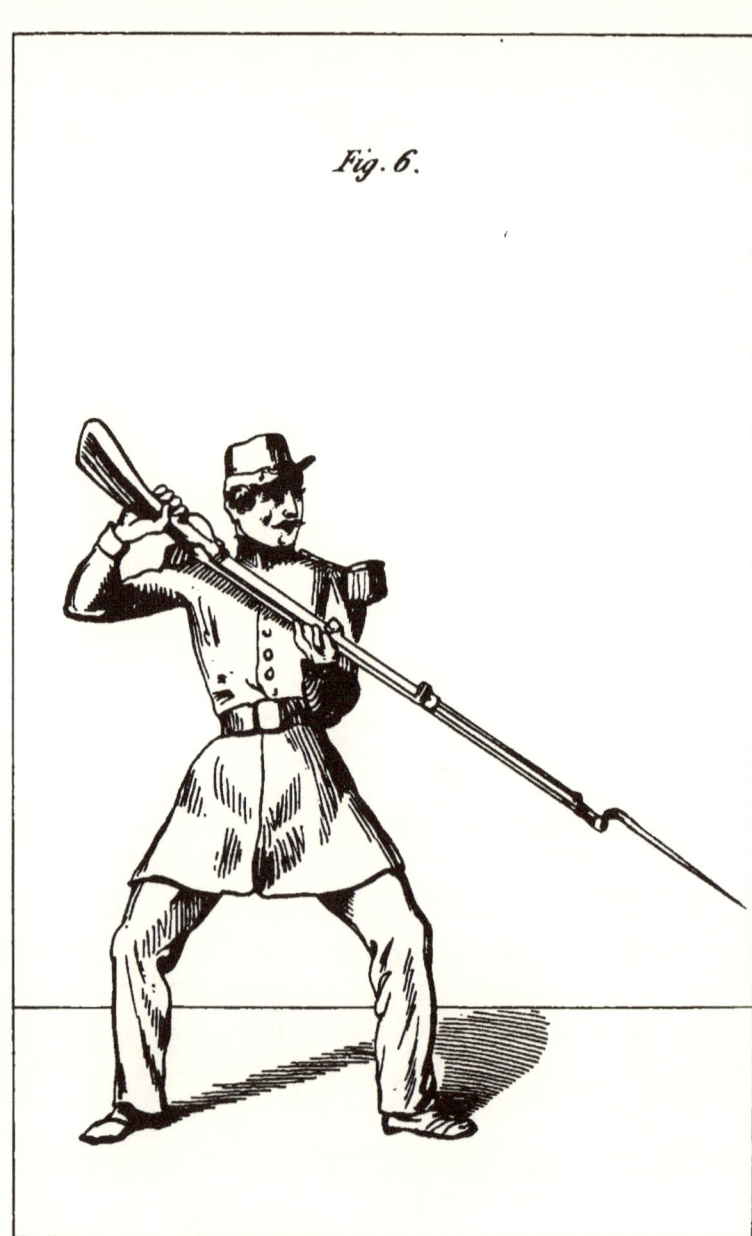

Fig. 6.

Parry two.

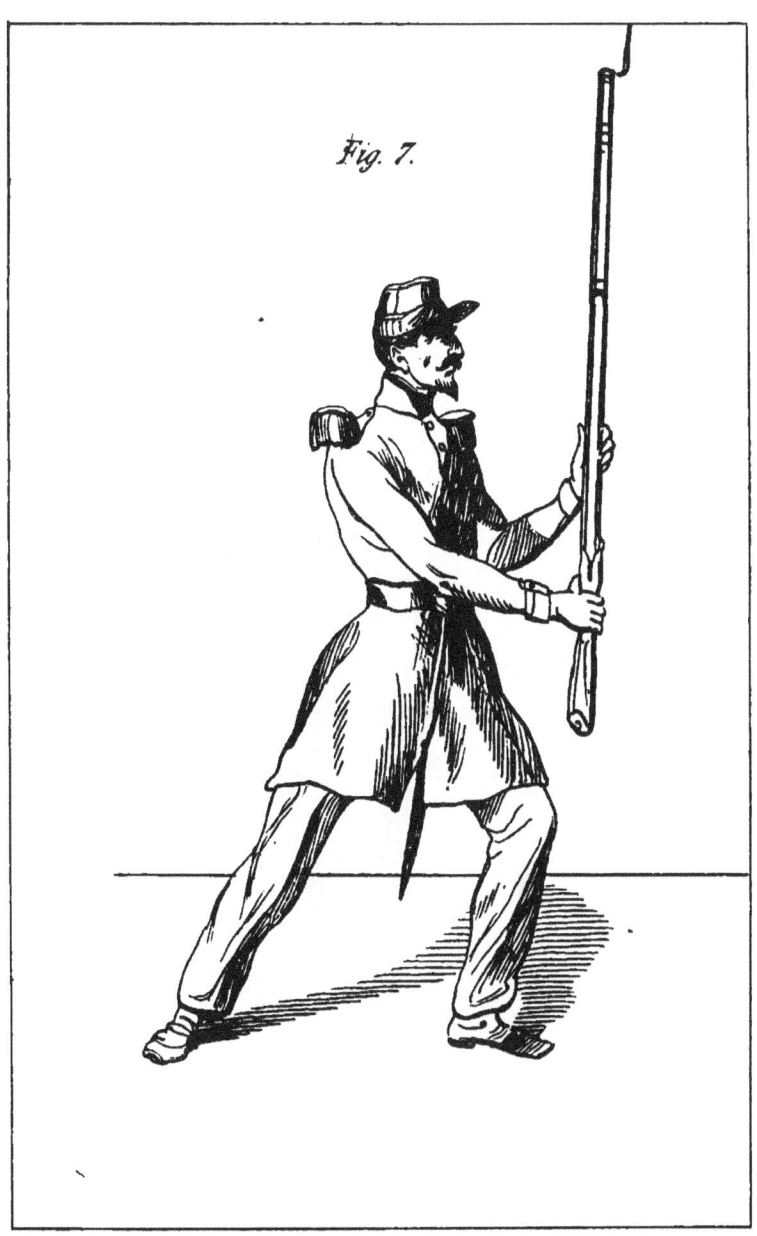

With the bull parry.

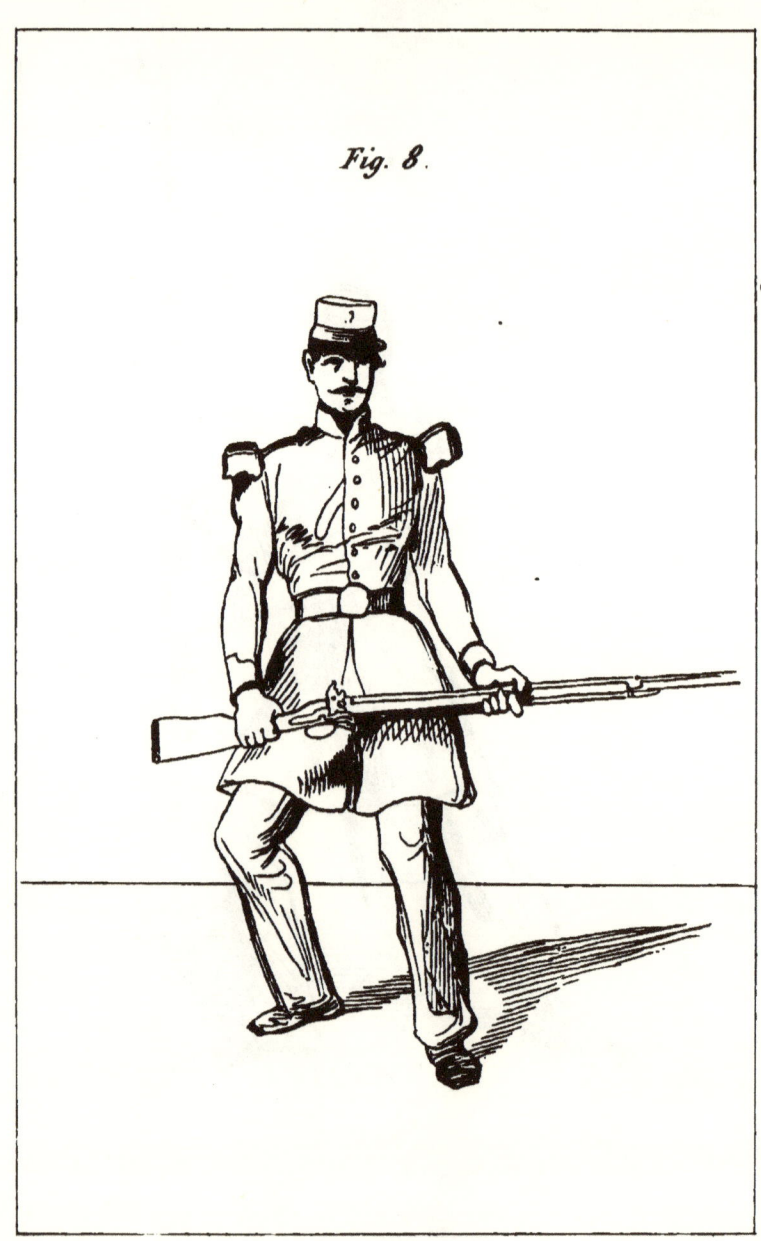

Body parry.

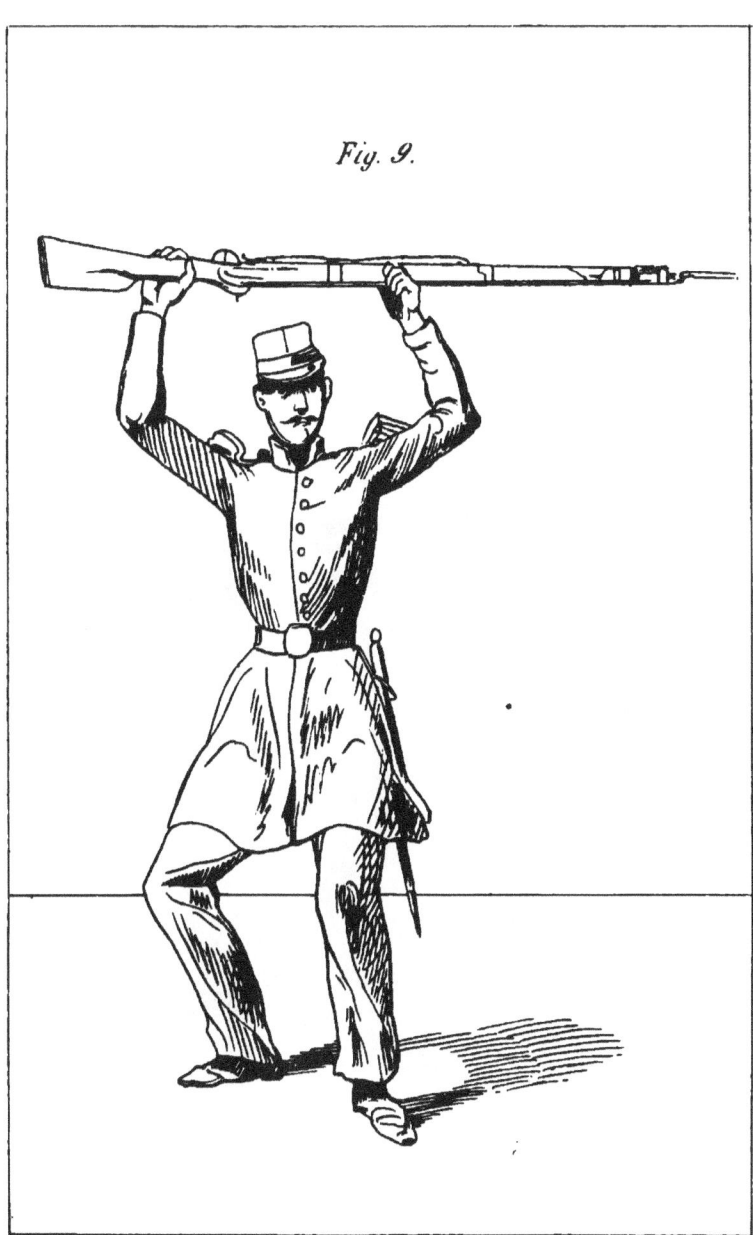

Fig. 9.

Head parry.

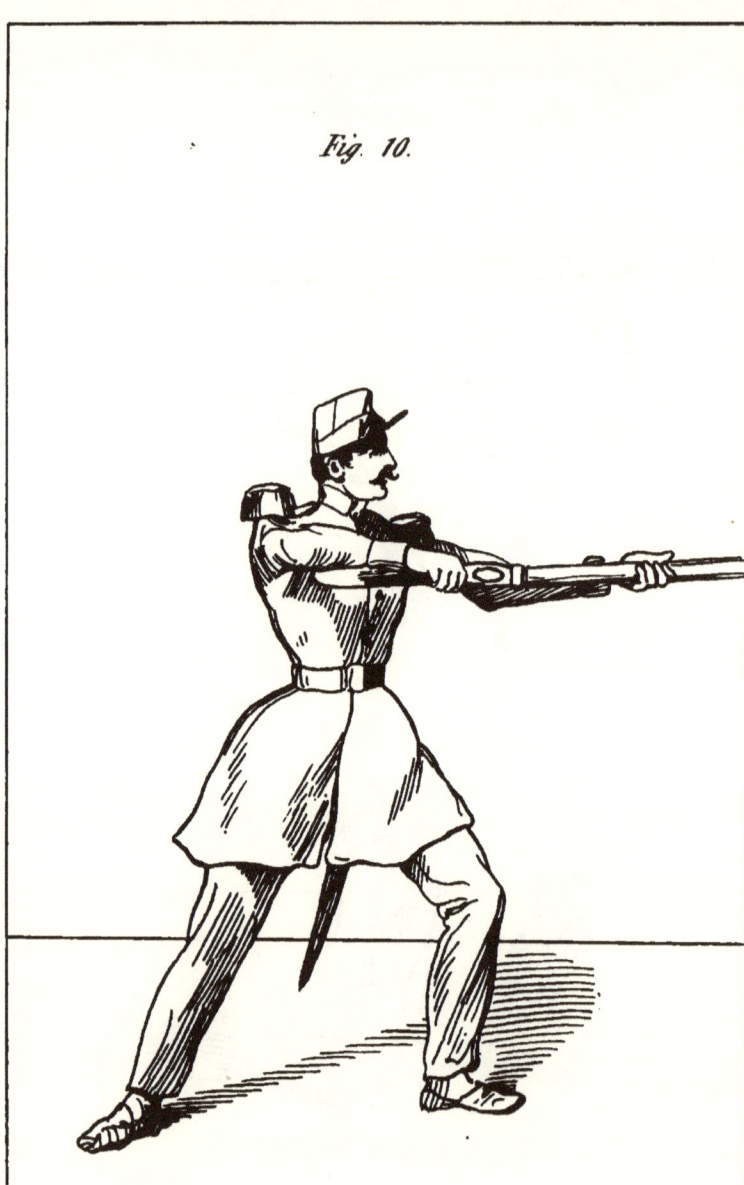

Lunge one.

Parry two—ARMS. (*Two motions.*) (Fig. 6.)

1. Turn rapidly the rammer upward; describe a half-circle with the point of the bayonet from above to below, to throw the piece of the adversary outside of the line of the right knee, without moving the left hand, the left elbow closed into and resting on the left breast, the right hand opposite the right shoulder at the height of the eye.
2. Resume guard. (The figure 6, represents the parry being executed, not completed.)

With the butt parry—ARMS. (*Four motions.*) (Fig. 7.)

1. Straighten the right leg; bring the gun perpendicularly before the centre of the body, the lock to the front, the right arm nearly straight, the thumb of the left hand not higher than the shoulder.
2. Move the butt of the piece to the left.
3. Move the butt of the piece to the right.
4. Resume guard.

Body and head parry—ARMS. (*Three motions.*) (Figs. 8 and 9.)

1. Bring the left hand near the left hip; advance the right hand; place the piece horizontally before the body, lowering it to the thighs, the barrel upward.
2. Raise it immediately just above the top of the cap, the barrel downward, the fingers of the left hand closed.
3. Resume guard.

THIRD LESSON.

LUNGES AND THRUSTS.

Lunge one—ARMS. (*Two motions.*) (Fig. 10.)

1. Bring rapidly the piece to a horizontal position (the lock plate up) in the direction of the breast of the adversary, by extending the left arm to its full length, the flat of the butt under the right forearm; strengthen the right leg, throwing forward the body.
2. Resume guard.

Lunge two—ARMS. (*Two motions.*) (Figs. 11 and 12.)

1. Draw the piece back with the right hand, the left hand following the piece in order to give it a greater impulse; direct quickly the bayonet towards the breast of the adversary, by extending the right arm, making the piece slide horizontally through the left hand up to the trigger guard, the lock upward, the flat of the butt under the right forearm, and the right leg straight.

2. Resume guard.

Lunge three—ARMS. (*One motion.*) (Fig. 13.)

Thrust quickly the piece against your adversary by a full extension of the right arm, turning the lock upward, the flat of the butt under the right forearm, the upper part of the body following the motion of the right hand, the left hand (which has quit its hold in making the lunge) open ready to receive the piece, and resume quickly the guard.

Thrust three—ARMS. (Fig. 14.)

Extend quickly the left arm, directing the point of the bayonet on the left breast of the adversary; raise the piece at the same time to the height of the face and within four inches of it, turning the trigger guard upwards, the butt resting upon the right forearm; straighten the right leg, the upper part of the body thrown forward.

2. Resume the guard.

Thrust four—ARMS. (Fig. 15.)

1. Direct quickly the point of the bayonet on the right breast of the adversary, the lock downward, the piece under the left arm, the butt-plate against the breast, the left arm extended, with the left hand holding the piece, the right hand remaining at the small of the stock, the right leg straight, the upper part of the body forward.

2. Resume the guard.

Thrust one—ARMS. (*Two motions.*)

1. Take the position of parry one, and thrust by ex-

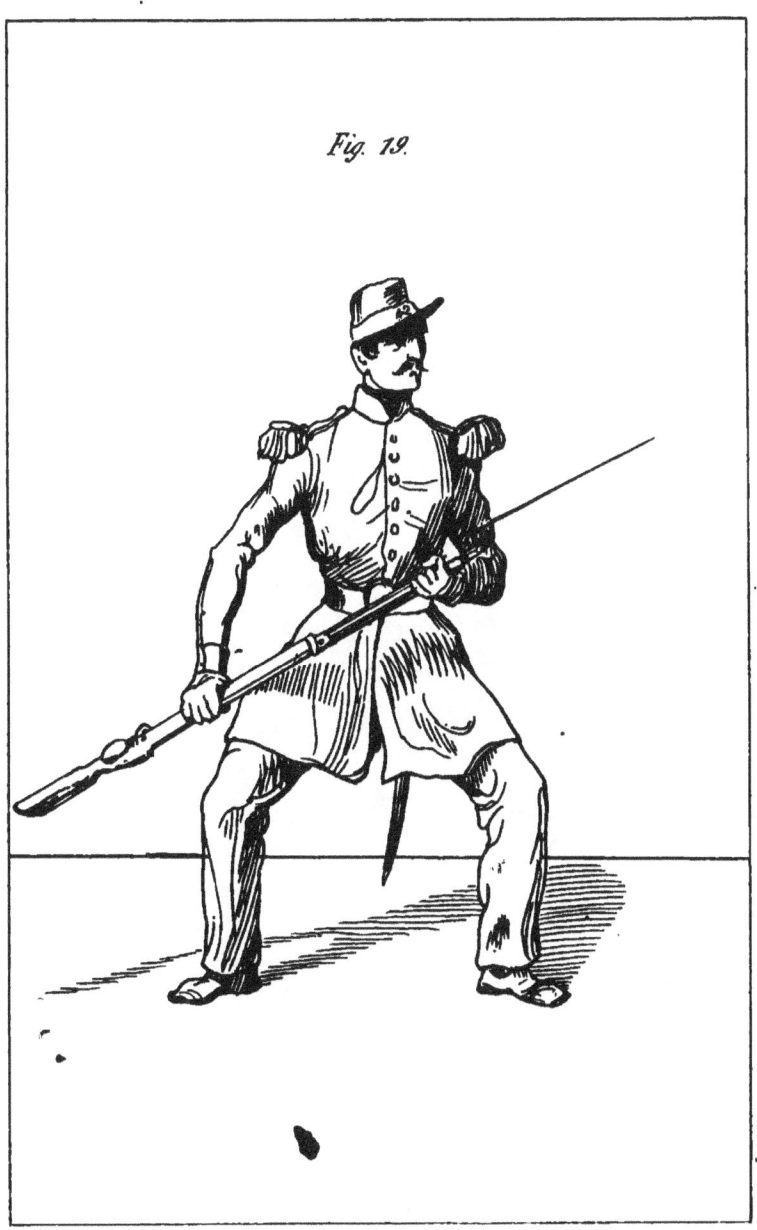

Preparation for shortened stroke.

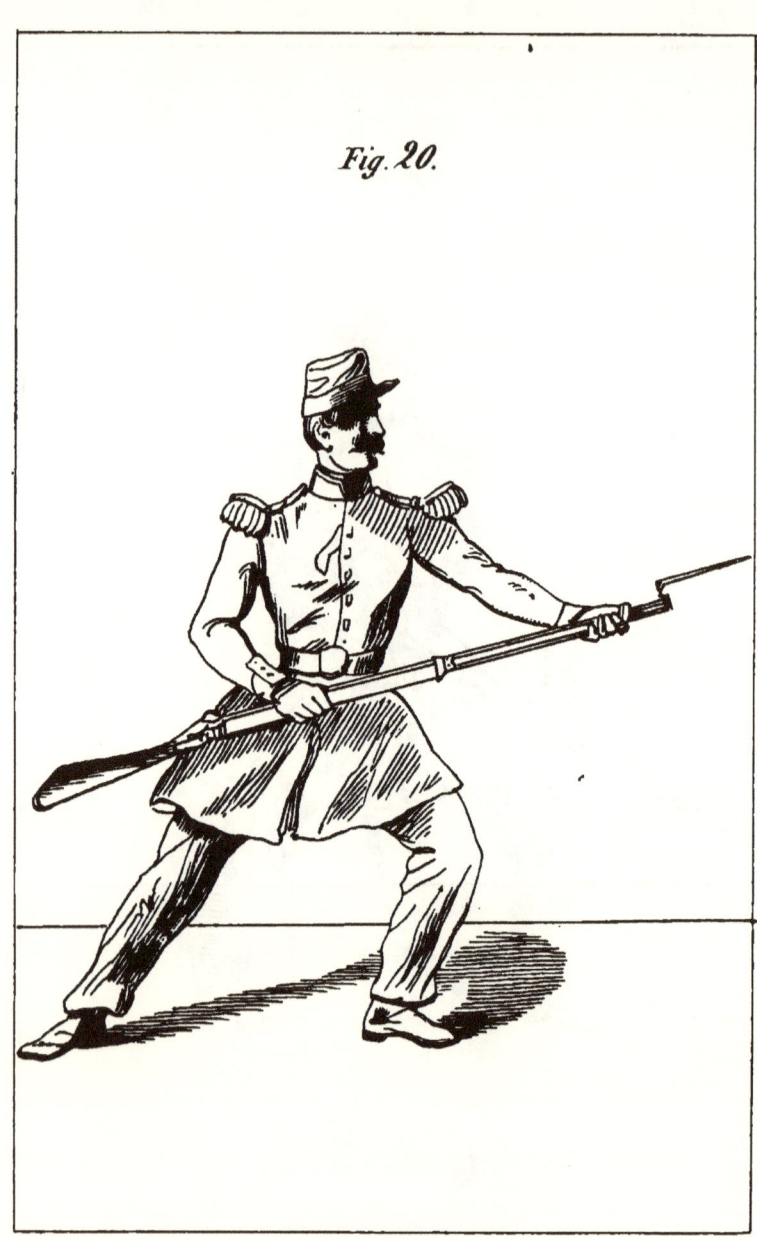

Fig. 20.

Shortened stroke.

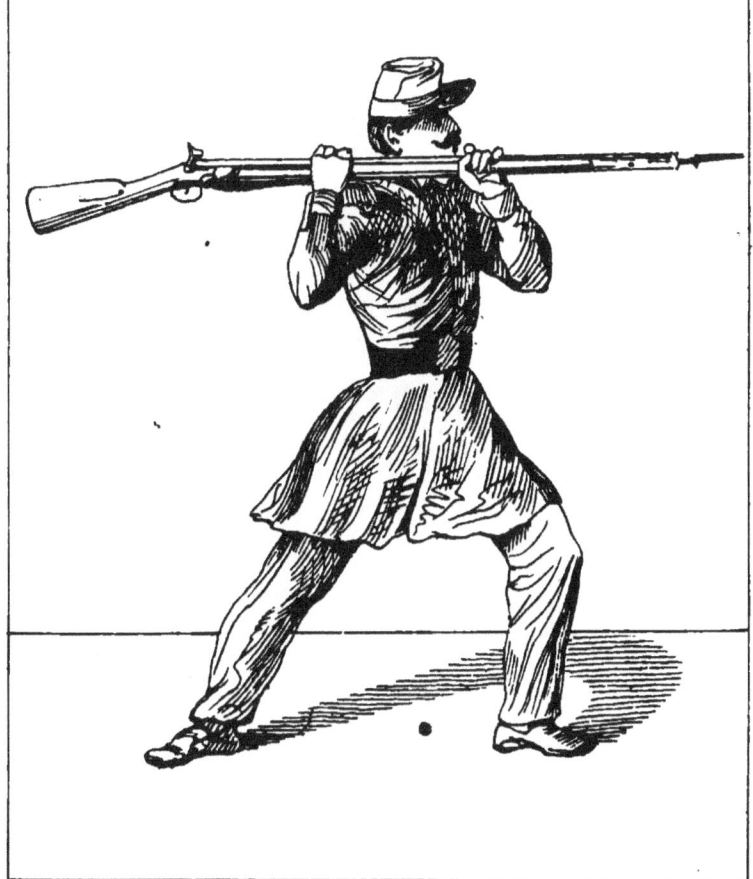

Fig. 21.

Coup de mêlée.

Fig. 22.

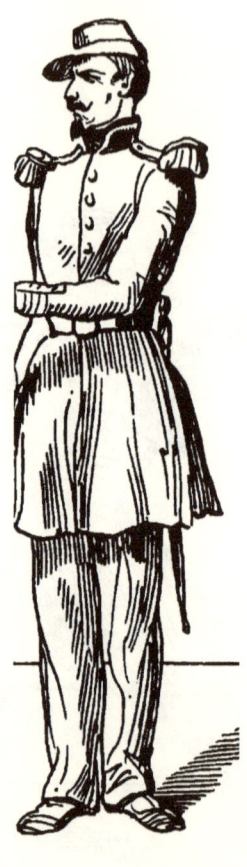

Salute to the right.

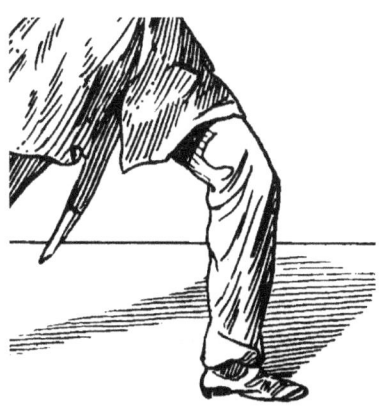

Thrust four.

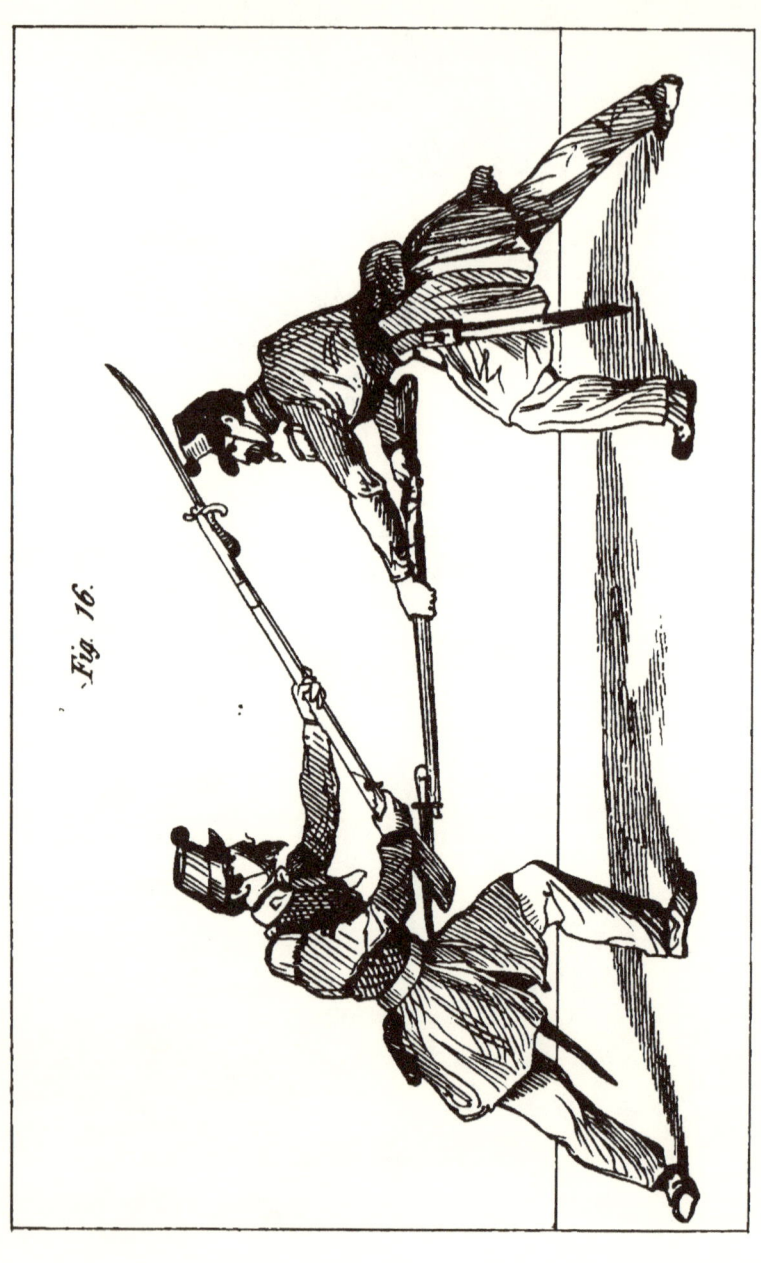
Fig. 16.

Fig. 17.

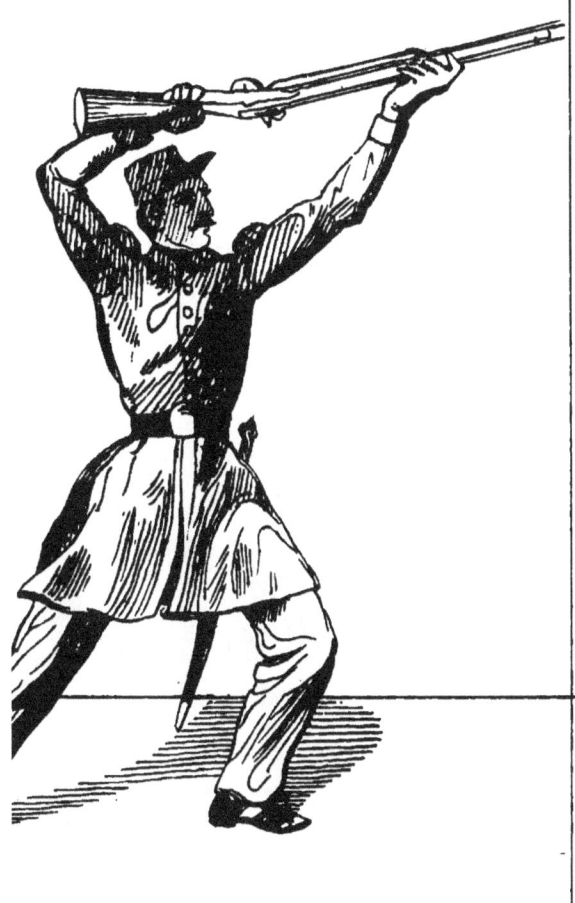

Thrust one against Cavalry.

Fig. 18.

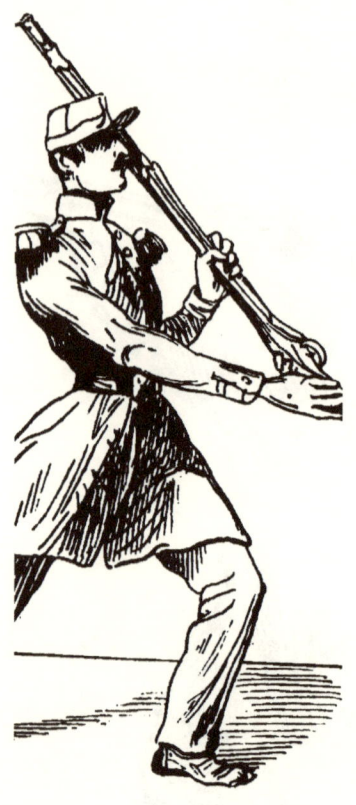

with the butt.

Fig. 19.

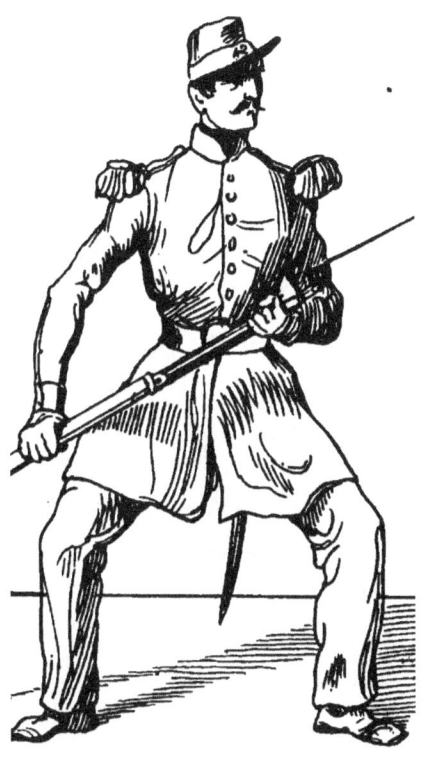

Preparation for shortened stroke.

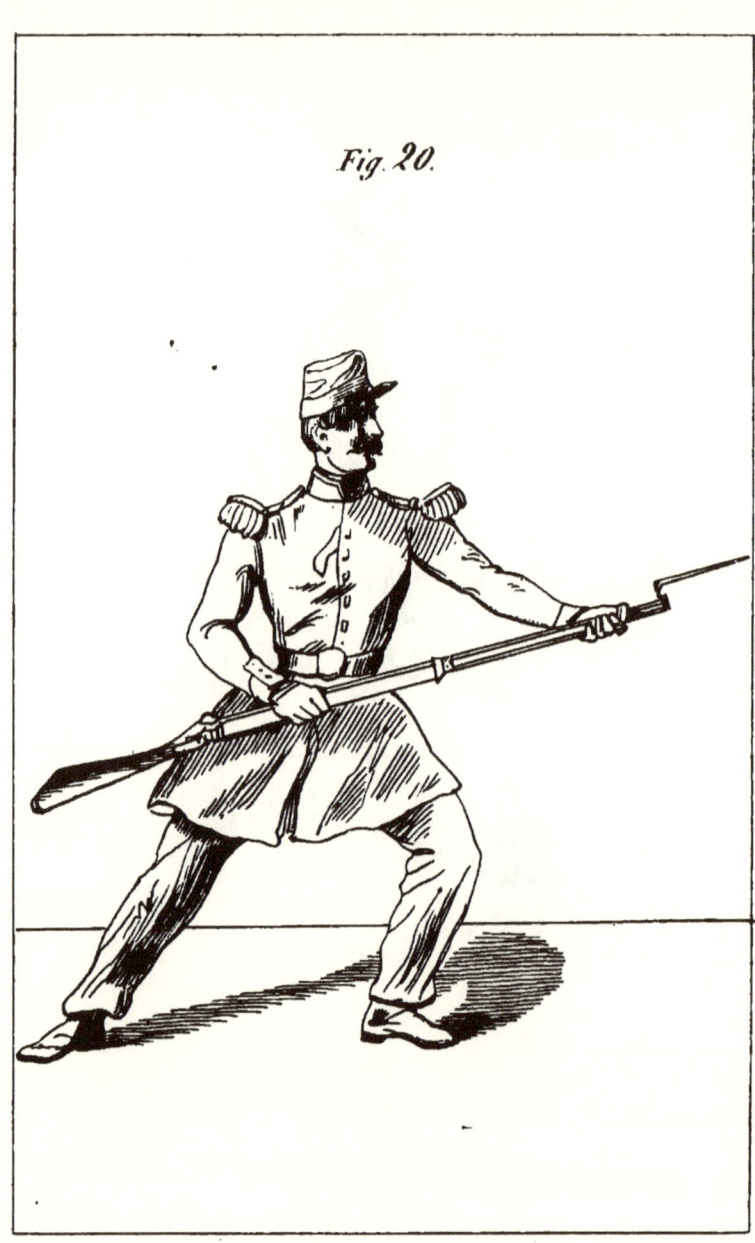

Fig. 20.

Shortened stroke.

Fig. 21.

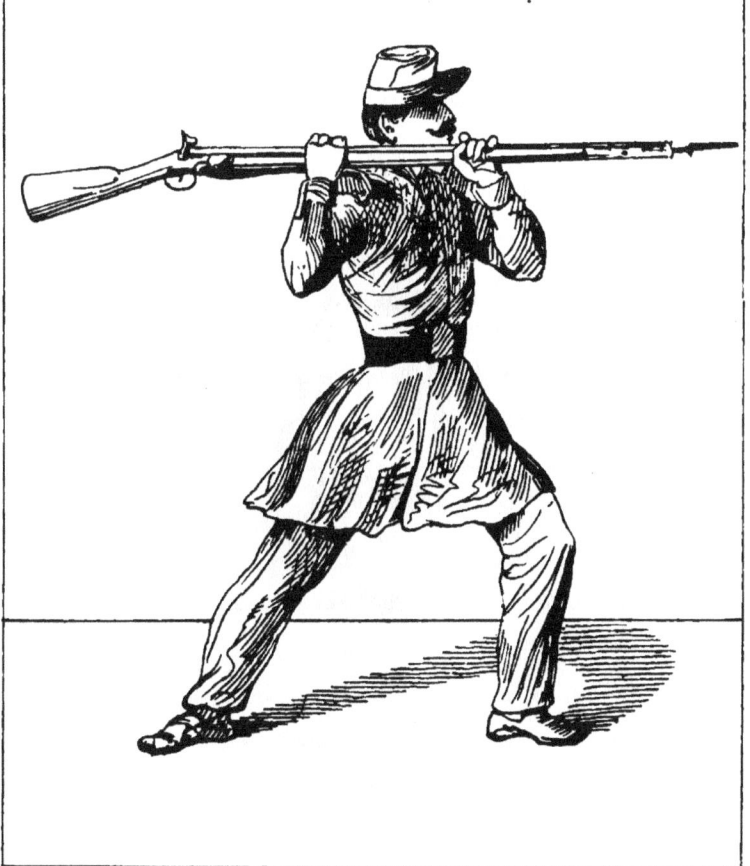

Coup de mêlée.

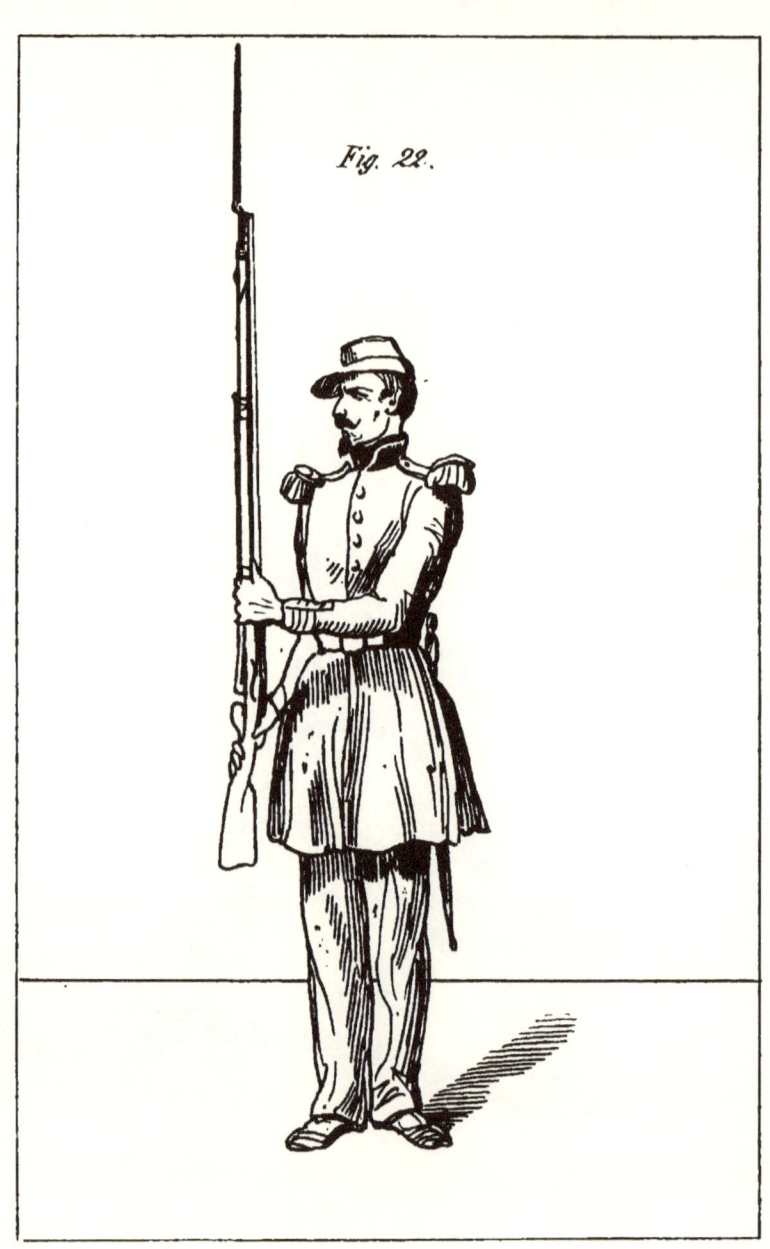

Salute to the right.

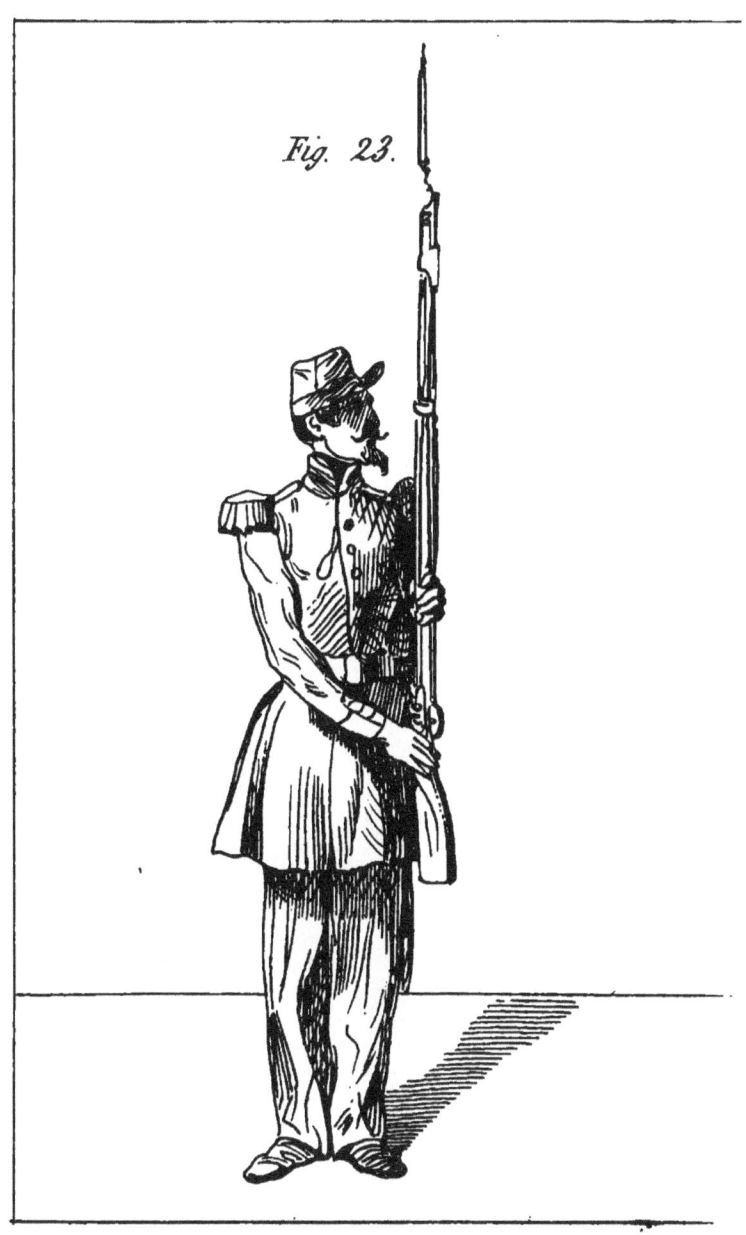

Salute to the left.

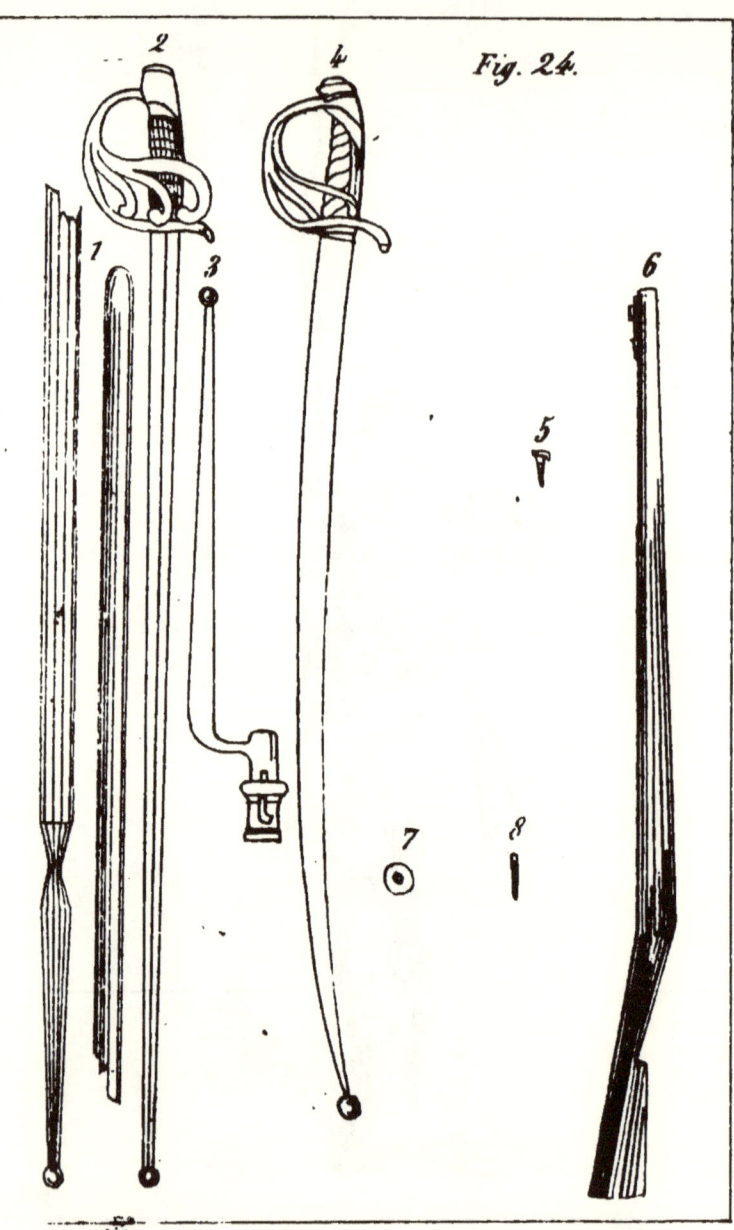

Fig. 24.

1. Lance.
2. Saber of heavy cavalry.
3. Bayonet in gutta-percha.
4. Saber of light cavalry.
5. Screw.
6. Wooden Gun.
7. Round piece of iron.
8. Pin to fasten the bayonet on the wooden gun.

tending the arms,—the point of the bayonet directed on the belly of your adversary, just below the belt.

2. Resume the guard.

(This thrust can be advantageously parried with the butt, and can be replied to by the thrust *four*, or a cut or blow, as shown in fig. 16.)

Thrust two—ARMS.

Take the position of parry two, and thrust by extending the arms as in thrust one.

Against cavalry, thrust—ONE. (Three motions.)
(Fig. 17.)

1. Raise the piece with both hands, the arms extended, the trigger guard upward, the hand between the thumb and fingers of the left hand.
2. Bend the left knee and straighten the right knee, thrusting at the height of a man on horseback.
3. Resume the guard.

AGAINST INFANTRY.

With the butt strike—ARMS. (Three motions.) (Fig. 18.)

1. Extend quickly the right arm to its full length, draw back the piece with the left to within five inches of the breast; straighten the right knee; strike the adversary in the lower part of the belly, with the toe of the butt.
2. Then on the head, with the barrel, by drawing back the right hand, using the left as a pivot.
3. Resume guard.

Shortened stroke—ARMS. (Three motions.)
(Figs. 19 and 20.)

1. Jerk the piece back with the left hand, which will be placed near the upper band, the left forearm touching the body, the right hand seizing the piece at the tail-band.
2. Straighten the right knee; extend quickly the left arm its full length in thrusting.
3. Resume the guard.

Coup de melée—ARMS.　　(*Three motions.*)　　(Fig. 21.)

1. Pitch up the piece with both hands to the height of the chin, and about three inches from it, seize it with right hand (the back of it turned outwards) at the tail-band, and with the left hand at the middle band, the back of it turned inwards.

2. Thrust, straightening the right knee, and bring back the piece—the right hand opposite the shoulder.

3. Give the piece a rotary motion in that hand (the right) with the left hand, which leaves the hold of the piece to seize it again in front of the right hand; place the latter at the small of the stock, resuming the guard.

FOURTH LESSON.

COMBINED MOTIONS, PARRIES AND THRUSTS, STANDING FAST.

3.	Parry three, and thrust			
3.	"	four,	"	"
3.	"	one,	"	"
3.	"	two,	"	"
4.	"	three and four,	thrust four	
4.	"	four and three,	"	three
4.	"	one and two,	"	two
4.	"	two and one,	"	one
4.	"	one and three,	"	three
4.	"	two and four,	"	four
4.	"	two and three,	"	three
6.	With butt parry, and strike			
6.	"	"	"	shorten stroke
3.	"	"	"	thrust four
6.	Body and head parry—Coup de melée			
3.	Head parry against cavalry—Thrust one			

} ARMS.

The figures indicate the number of motions in executing the commands to which they are prefixed.

FIFTH LESSON.

In this lesson, which is preparatory instruction to the sixth, one must proceed after the following principles.

BAYONET EXERCISE.

The thrusts are delivered standing fast, and after a motion forward. The parries are made when standing fast, and after a motion backward. One may execute, indifferently, either a thrust or a parry after the following motions: Right or left face. Right about or left about face. A pace to the right or to the left. The commands relating to the legs, must always precede those relating to the arms. A command must include only one motion of the legs with one thrust or one parry, as—

Extend—lunge one,	March.	(2 motions.)
One pace forward—lunge two,	"	4 "
" " backward—parry one,	"	4 "
Passade forward—lunge three,	"	4 "
" backward—with butt parry,	"	6 "
" forward, against cavalry—parry one,	"	3 "
*Leap to the rear—parry two,	"	2 "
* " " head and body parry,	"	4 "

SIXTH LESSON.

MOVEMENTS FORWARD---THRUSTS AND PARRIES.
MOVEMENTS BACKWARD---PARRIES AND THRUSTS.

† Extend, lunge one, parry three,	March.	(3 motions.)
One pace forward, lunge two, parry four,	"	5 "
" backward, parry four and thrust four,	"	5 "
Passade forward, parry three (or four), shorten stroke,	"	6 "
" backward, with butt parry, and strike,	"	8 "
" backward, with butt parry, shorten stroke,	"	8 "
" backward, with butt parry, thrust four,	"	7. "

---

* To parry with the leap, the parry is made at the same time with the leap.

† The lunge is made in the same time with the extension, and the parry in the same time, and when in the act of resuming guard.

Passade forward, against cavalry,
 thrust one, head parry, March. (5 motions.)
Leap to the rear, parry two, thrust
 two, . " 3 "
 " " body and head parry, •
  Coup de melée, " 7 "

After the motions, face to the right or left, right or left about face, one pace to the right or to the left, one can execute indifferently the thrusts and parries or the parries and thrusts of this lesson.

BAYONET EXERCISE,

WITH THE RIFLE AND SABRE BAYONET.

1. In teaching this exercise, the men will be placed in one rank, at a distance of four paces from each other, in order that they may not be able to meet when vaulting.

2. The men being at a light infantry shoulder, the instructor will command:

    1. *Guard against Infantry* (Pl. 1).
    2. GUARD. (Two motions.)

3. 1st motion: Make a half-face to the right on both heels, the feet square; raise at the same time the piece a little, and seize it with the left hand below and near the middle band.

4. 2d motion: Bring the right leg to the rear perpendicularly, about eighteen inches, the right heel on the same line with the left; the knees a little bent, the weight of the body bearing equally on both legs; lower the piece with both hands, the barrel upward, the left elbow pressing against the body; seize at the same time the piece below the trigger-guard with the right hand; the arms hanging naturally, the point of the bayonet slightly elevated.

    Shoulder—ARMS. (One motion.)

5. Raise the piece with the left hand; place it against the right shoulder; bring at the same time the right heel on the alignment of the left, and face to the front.

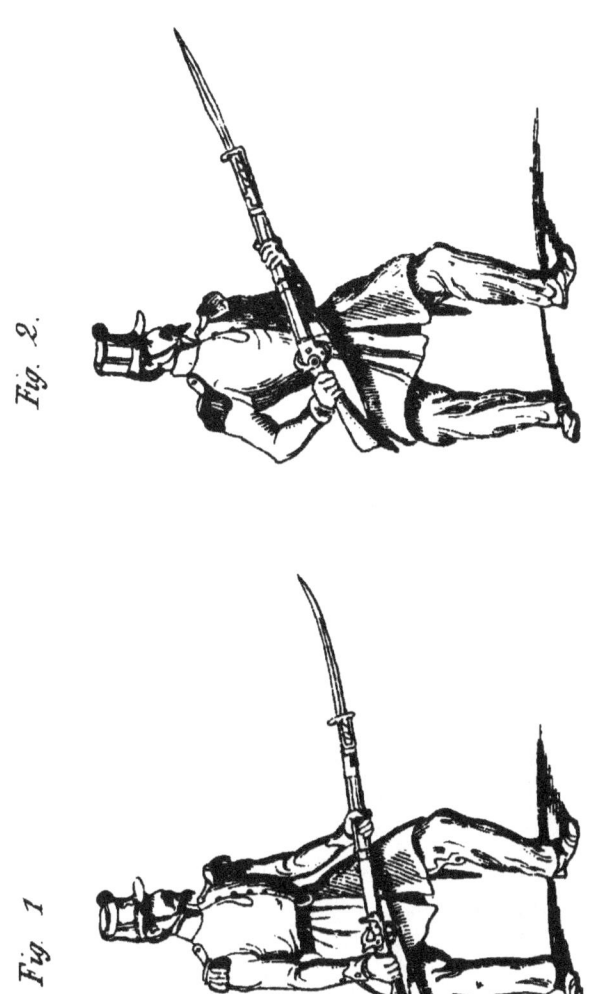

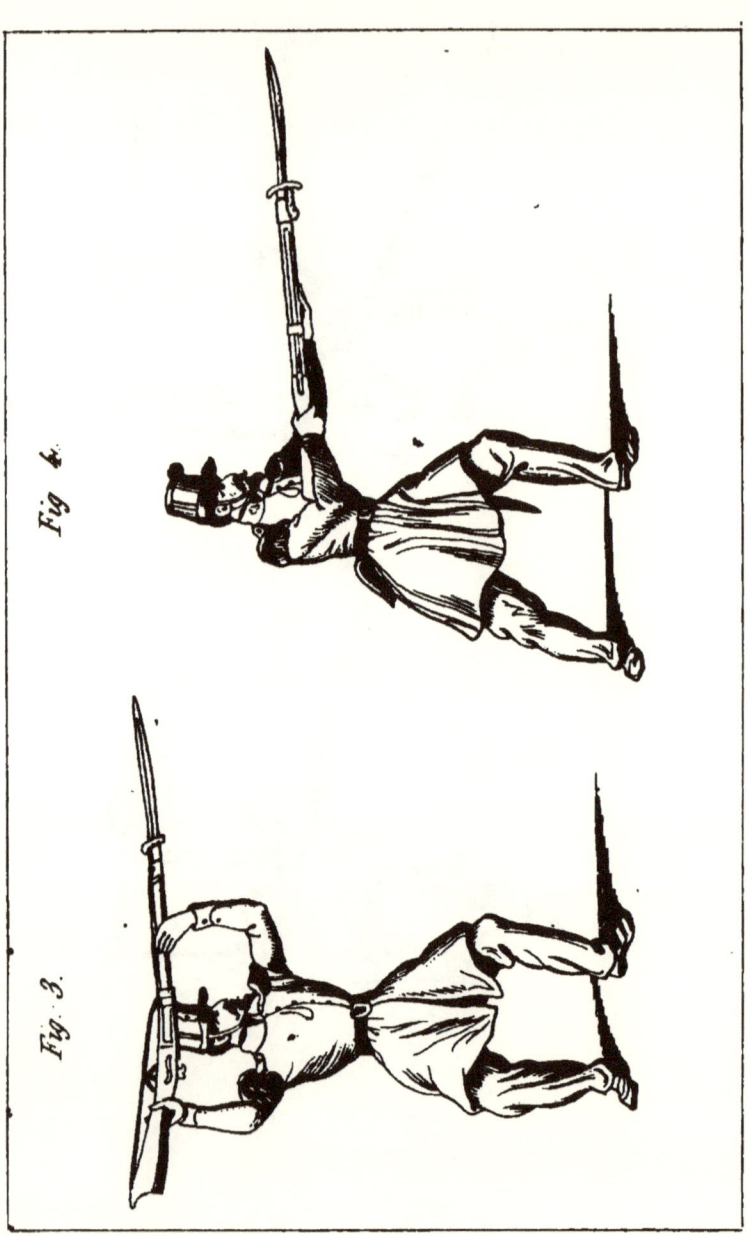

1. *Guard against Cavalry.* (Pl. 2.)
2. GUARD. (Two motions.)

6. The first and the second motions as in the guard against infantry, with the exception that the right hand will be fixed at the hip, and the bayonet as high as the eye, as in the position of charge bayonet.

7. The men placed in either of the above positions, will execute the following motions:

1. *Face to the right (or left).*
2. *Right (or left)*—FACE.

8. Turn on the left heel, by raising the toe, and face to the right (or left); at the same time bring the right foot to the rear, at eighteen inches.

1. *Face to the right about.*
2. *Right about*—FACE.

9. At the command *face*, turn to the right on the left heel, by raising the toe a little; face to the rear without changing the position of the piece, and bring the right foot to the rear, at eighteen inches from the left.

1. *Face to the left about.*
2. *Left about*—FACE.

10. Turn to the left on the left heel by the inverse means of that above prescribed.

1. *One pace forward.* 2. MARCH.

11. At the command *march*, carry first the right foot against the left heel, and then the left foot at eighteen inches to the front.

1. *One pace backward.* 2. MARCH.

12. At the command *march*, carry first the left foot close to the right, and then the latter at eighteen inches to the rear.

1. *One pace to the right.* 2. MARCH.

13. Carry the right foot eighteen inches to the right in the same direction; bring immediately the left foot in front, at its distance, and in its position.

1. *One pace to the left.* 2. MARCH.

14. Carry the left foot eighteen inches to the left; bring immediately the right foot at its distance and in its position.

1. *Passade forward.* 2. MARCH.

15. Carry the right foot eighteen inches in front of the left; bring quickly the left foot eighteen inches in front, and preserve the position of the guard.

1. *Passade backward.* 2. MARCH.

16. Carry the left foot twelve inches in the rear of the right; bring quickly the right foot eighteen inches in the rear of the left; preserve the position of the guard.

1. *Volt to the right.* 2. MARCH.

17. Bring the piece near the body with the left hand, the barrel opposite the left shoulder, without moving the right hand; turn to the right on the toe of the right foot, planting the left foot perpendicularly to the rear at eighteen inches; finish the volt by turning the toe of the left foot, and bringing the right foot to the rear and at its distance; resume the guard at the same time.

1. *Volt to the left.* 2. MARCH.

18. Turn to the left on the toe of the right foot; plant the left foot perpendicularly to the rear, at eighteen inches; and finish the volt by inverse means of that above prescribed.

19. When the men, at home in those different positions, will be able to execute with precision and quickness the divers paces and volts, they will be taught the use of their weapon for attack and defence.

1. *In carte parry.* 2. ARMS.

20. At the 2d command, raise the muzzle of the piece twelve inches with the left hand, without moving the right; at the same time move the piece about six inches to the left, and remain in that position.

Resume Guard.

21. Lower quickly the left hand, without moving the right, and bring the piece to the position of the guard.

22. Each time the instructor causes the parries and the thrusts to be executed, he will cause the guard to be resumed at the end of each motion, by the command, *resume guard.*

1. *In tierce parry.* 2. ARMS.

23. Raise quickly the muzzle of the piece twelve inches with the left hand, without moving the right; at the same time move the piece with the left hand six inches to the right.

1. *In prime parry.* 2. ARMS. (Pl. 3.)

24. Raise the piece with both hands, the arms fully extended, the piece covering the head, the lock plate turned towards the body, the barrel grasped by the thumb and forefinger of the left hand, the bayonet menacing, although slightly inclined to the left, the tail-band at the top of the hat.

1. *In prime right (or left) parry.* 2. ARMS.

25. Advance the left shoulder (or the right shoulder) and parry (as explained in 24) to the right (or to the left.)

1. *In carte thrust.* 2. ARMS. (Pl. 4.)

26. At the second command, throw the weight of the body forward; bend the left knee and straighten the right; extend the left arm in full, the fingers of the left hand being open and maintaining the piece; bringing the butt before the left breast, the lock-plate turned downward; and remain in that position until the command *resume guard.*

1. *In tierce thrust.* 2. ARMS. (Pl. 5.)

27. Bring the upper part of the body forward; straighten the right knee and bend the left; fully extend the left arm, the fingers of the left hand being open and maintaining the piece, the lock-plate turned upward, the butt before the right breast.

1. *In prime thrust.* 2. ARMS. (Pl. 6.)

28. Elevate the piece with both hands, the arms being extended, the trigger-guard upward, the barrel between

the thumb and fingers of the left hand; bend the left knee and straighten the right, thrust at the same time the piece to the adversary, directing the blow at the height of a man on horseback.

 1. *In prime to the right (or left) thrust.*
 2. ARMS.

29. Advance the left shoulder (or the right shoulder) and thrust to the right (or to the left) as explained in 28.

 1. *Lunge.* 2. ARMS. (Pl. 7.)

30. At the 2d command, throw the upper part of the body forward, by bending the left knee and straightening the right; thrust rapidly the piece at the adversary, fully extending the right arm, leaving off with the left hand when thrusting, which is kept extended to receive the piece, and resume the guard.

31. When the men are on guard against infantry, they will thrust at the height of the breast of a man; when on guard against cavalry, they will aim the blow at the height of a horse's head, or of the sides of a horseman.

32. When the men are perfectly acquainted with the divers paces, parries, and thrusts, the instructor will cause them to execute those divers motions put together, at the command *march*. Example:

 1. *Passade forward, in prime parry and thrust.*
 2. MARCH.

33. At the 2d command, the man will execute the passade, parry in prime, and thrust in prime.

34. As one must admit the case when one single man will be in the necessity of defending himself against two or three adversaries, the instructor will cause the double motions and thrusts to be executed, and that will add considerably to the address and nimbleness of the men. Example:

 1. *One pace forward, lunge, volt to the left, in carte parry and thrust.* 2. MARCH.

35. At the 2d command, march forward, lunge, then execute the volt, parry carte, and thrust carte.

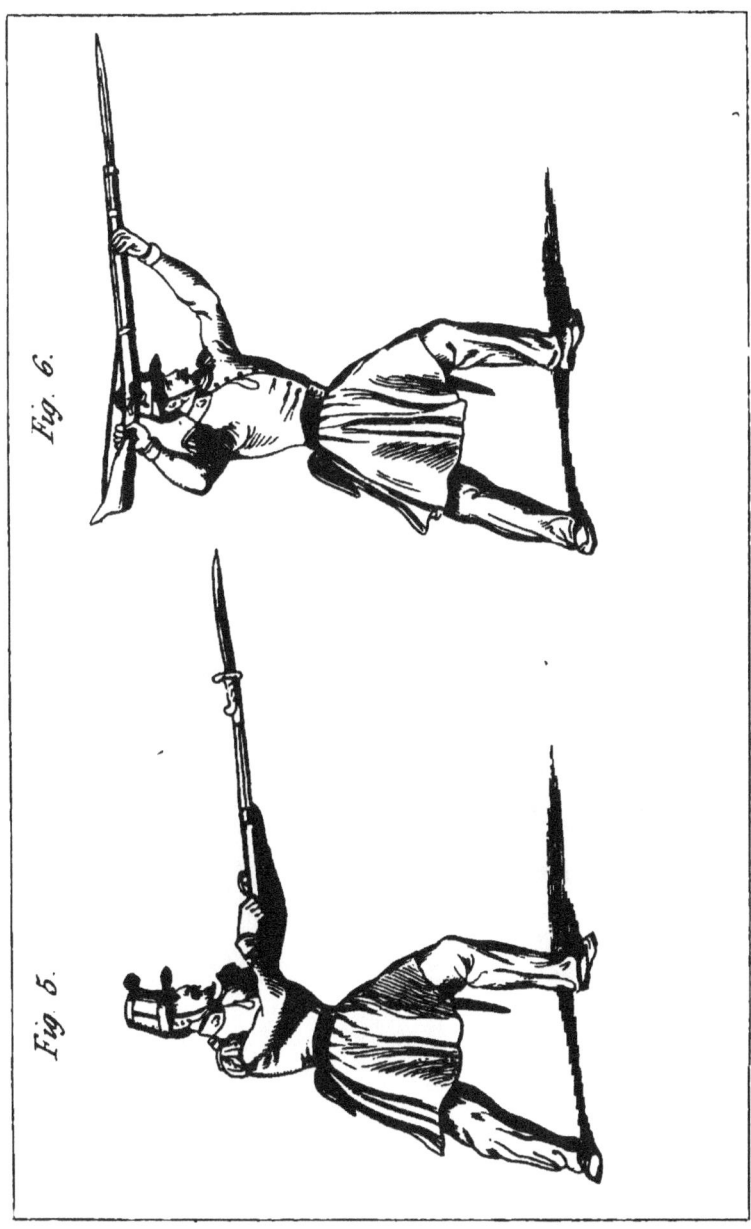

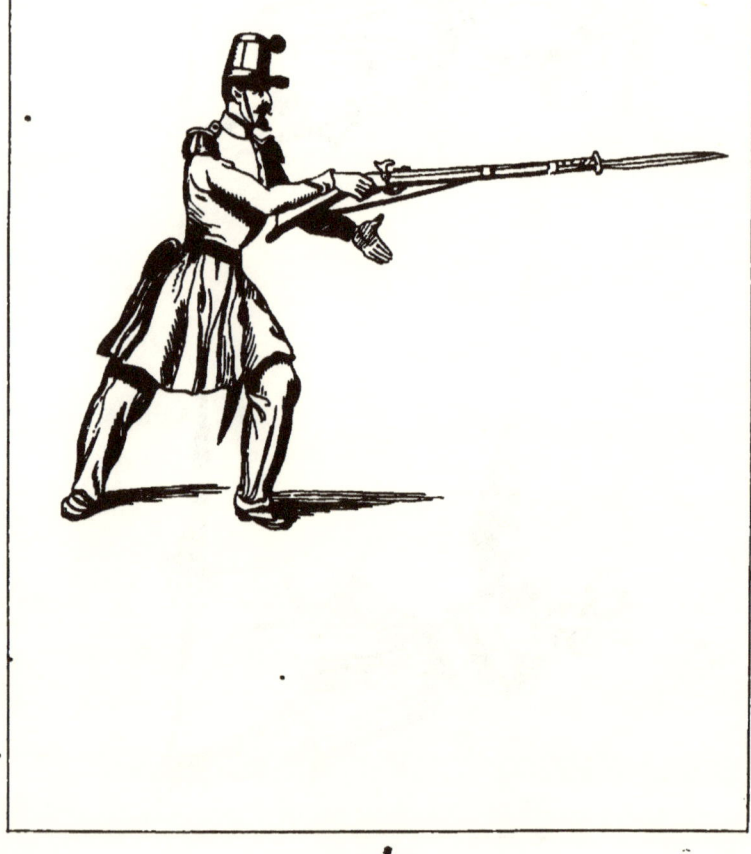

Lunge.

EXERCISE WITH THE PLASTRON.

In the lesson with the plastron, the same progression is followed as in the figurative lesson.

In order to obtain more rapidity in the execution of the motions, the pace forward and the pace backward will be executed on the command, *advance, retreat;* as for the other motions of the arms and legs, the commands *arms* and *march* are suppressed.

After the parries have been executed separately they will be executed by two, three, four, five, and six, together.

In the lesson with the plastron, the *Extension*, (fig. 2) always accompanies the lunge one, the lunge two, the thrusts three, four, one, and two.

The blows with the butt and the shortened stroke are generally delivered standing fast, and after a parry.

When the shortened stroke is used it must be repeated three times. One must not return the lunges one, two, or three, after the parry four or the parry one, except when the bayonet of the adversary has been well thrown off the line of carte, (the left side of the body); otherwise one is exposed to receive a blow at the same time.

The lunge three is not to be used against an infantry soldier, except with the greatest circumspection, because it leaves, when parried, the man at the mercy of his adversary; never "extend" when delivering it.

When the blow with the butt is delivered after parry three, the bayonet must pass over the right shoulder; on the contrary, it must pass over the left shoulder, if after parry four.

Salute. (Figs. 22 and 23.)

When two men are about to proceed to a fencing-match, the salute will be made in the following manner: Being at a light infantry carry, take the guard, and engage the end of the bayonet in carte; make two appeals,—that is, strike the ground twice, smartly, with the left foot,—and immediately after take the erect position, by bringing the right heel against the left, so that the feet be square to each other; raise at the same time the piece against the right shoulder, the left arm on the breast, the hand at the height of the shoulder; salute to the right by presenting the piece towards that side,—that is to say, by turning the ramrod to the right, the piece being perpendicular opposite to the shoulder; turn, also, the head to the right; salute to the left by similar motions of the piece and head; bring back the piece opposite the middle of the body to salute the adversary by lowering, a little, both hands; resume the guard; make two "appeals;" then the fencing begins.

Materiel. (Fig. 24.)

The materiel in the fencing-room should consist of plastrons of buckskin, masks and gloves, as for fencing with the broadsword (the left hand only should require a glove); muskets made of ash or hickory, and gutta percha bayonets; also, a lance and a sabre, prepared as the bayonet, to be used in sham-fights against a horseman.

SUGGESTIONS FOR THE SOLDIER IN A FIGHT.

HOW TO FIGHT A FOOT SOLDIER.

When the bayonets are engaged for a fight, if your adversary succeeds, by means of a strong pressure, to move your piece towards the right or left, it will be necessary then to yield to that pressure in such a manner as to parry one or two; if, for instance, the pressure is felt towards the left, yield in the same manner, parry two and thrust two, and return to the position of parry one, or parry two, according to circumstances. When attacked by two infantry soldiers marching without interval between them, wait for them in front in a defensive attitude, and, as soon as they are within reach, deliver lunge three and pass to the right, if the lunge is delivered against the man on the left; by inverse means one should pass to the left, if the lunge was delivered against the man on the right. If the blow has taken effect, the fight will be continued with the next man; but, admitting that the lunge was parried by the former, the motion of passing to the right (or left) has brought you to the right (or left) flank, and given you time for new thrusts against your adversary, as the other man, until he has also shifted his position, is masked by the one you have engaged.

If the two adversaries are advancing with an interval between them, with the view of attacking by the flanks and placing you between them, rush diagonally against the man on your right, or that on your left, attack him vigorously, and force him to turn his back to the other man when facing you. If the two adversaries are advancing in order to close upon you, the one in front, the other in the rear, then run to meet one of them in order to attack him and to turn him, as above.

In a crowd, use the *coup de melée;* and against several adversaries, with room enough for fencing, take the guard of *parry two* or *parry one*, and make volts, delivering a thrust each time you turn.

How to Fight a Horseman.

The strength of a horseman lies in his individual address and audacity much more than in his arms, which are little to be feared by a man skilled in the use of the bayonet. A wary horseman is careful not to approach an infantry man as long as the foot-soldier has a load in his gun. He will ride about, at a distance of a hundred paces or more, and fire with pistols or carbine, in order to draw the fire of the foot-soldier. In such a case the foot-soldier will take his aim at the horseman at the instant the horseman is firing, and go through the motions of taking cartridge, priming, &c., in order to induce the belief that his piece is not loaded.

The infantry soldier who is a good shot, and, at the same time, a good *bayonetsman*, waits, standing fast, for the horseman who charges him. He takes aim at his adversary, and fires as soon as the latter is within six or eight yards distance; immediately after firing he takes the left of the horseman, if he does not already occupy that position. The footman must always manage to occupy that position, which is the least advantageous to the horseman, who has less facility for handling his sabre to his left than to his right. A dead-shot aims at the man; an ordinary shot aims at the horse, and runs up to the horseman as he falls; and the defeat of the horseman is then an easy matter.

However, a man nimble and confident in his weapon, although taking aim at his adversary, holds his fire. He uses first his bayonet, and only fires when the horseman has passed him, or even later, when he thinks it necessary to bring the fight to an end.

If the horseman is armed with a sabre, he cannot reach further than two yards, and the infantry soldier, by placing himself at that distance, only looks for an opportunity of delivering the lunge three, by means of which he is able to reach the horseman at a distance of three yards. If the horseman manages to get near enough to the man to have him within reach of his sabre, then the infantry soldier will parry three and four by presenting his piece vertically, and taking care to lower the piece, and to protect the fingers of his left hand behind the barrel. He takes the guard of head parry (fig. 9), and returns by the thrust against cavalry (fig. 17), or by the lunge three, which is used principally against cavalry.

When the horseman is armed with a lance, the two adversaries can reach from the same distance. The foot-soldier will avoid the first shock, or any blow which participates in the momentum acquired by the impulsion of the horse; whether he happens to be placed to the left or to the right, he must, when parrying, throw his piece in the direction of the motion of the horse. When he has succeeded in warding off the blow of his adversary, he closes as quickly as possible, if the horseman keeps circling around him, and multiplies his attacks with the bayonet. The lancer, in close quarters, finds great difficulty in parrying and thrusting. A skillful horseman, who can cause the infantry soldier to lose his self-possesion (*sang froid*), will have the advantage of him; but, if the latter keeps cool, with his gun loaded, he will be able to conquer one, and even two horsemen.

A foot-soldier who has been engaged in or witnessed a fight with a horseman, is soon convinced of the superiority of his means, and cannot be scared by the impetuous charge of his adversary.

If the horseman comes direct upon the infantry soldier, the latter will deliver the lunge three on the mouth of the horse, and make a step to the right, parrying four at the same time, if the horseman be armed with a sabre; on the contrary, he will pass to the left, if the horseman be a lancer, and parry three; returning the thrust one against cavalry (fig. 17), if the adversary is near enough, and lunge three, if not.

The most critical position for the foot-soldier is that in which he finds himself opposed to a skillful adversary, who will charge him impetuously in front, and suddenly oblique to the left, at a distance of ten paces, then oblique to the right again, in order to keep his man on his right. This circular motion has a tendency to bewilder the footman and make him dizzy. The foot-soldier will then take his stand at nine feet from the horseman, parry three and four, making paces to the right and lunging three whenever an opportunity occurs.

If the foot-soldier wishes to get out of the circle in which the trooper has placed him, he will direct himself by the shortest way to the rear of the horseman, and lunge three against the sides of the man or the horse.

If the horseman comes out unhurt, and makes to the right, taking a circuitous road, in order to keep again the foot soldier to his right, go straight to the front of the trooper, and strike the head of the horse.

If the trooper, instead of taking a roundabout way, makes right about face, in order to sabre the foot-soldier on his right, one must, in such a case, close at once with the horseman, from behind and at his left; and that ought to be done at the instant that the trooper slackens the motion of his horse in order to right about face. As soon as the foot-soldier has closed on the left, he will lunge three on the left side of the horseman.

Against two horsemen, the fencing will be carried on according to the same principles as against two infantry soldiers. It is hardly necessary to repeat that composure of mind, coolness, and resolution, are the requisites, in such encounters, in order to insure success.

www.ingramcontent.com/pod-product-compliance
Lightning Source LLC
Chambersburg PA
CBHW020337090426
42735CB00009B/1573